"Harley has succeeded in demystifiying the secret to good health and fitness . . . and it's no magic trick. Armed with a vast understanding of physiology and body mechanics, Harley has developed an exercise program that is intense yet remarkably simple; one that proves anyone can get results they want in less time and with greater efficiency."

—Benjamin Bratt

"I used to spend hours a week on weight training, but Harley taught me how to get better results in just twenty-five minutes a day, five days a weeks."

—Christian Slater

"Working with Harley was an incredible asset to my performance in *Cold Creek Manor*, our first of many films together. The cardio training meets the weight training was a terrific blend of training and the results were overwhelming. He made it fun which it never has been for me and I believe for most people."

—Stephen Dorff

"When you get down to it, you only need to look at Harley to understand that his system totally works. He's a permanent example of what to do to look fit."

—Lambert Wilson

"It isn't easy training someone who doesn't like to be told what to do. I am as stubborn as can be!! Given the parameters of my life and responsibilities, Harley cleverly managed to create an efficient and realistic workout that produced the promised results."

—Eliza Dushku

. . . *continued*

"Before I met Harley, I was never able to find the time or motivation to work out. Harley's brilliant regime of twenty-five minute workouts has enabled me to make fitness a part of my life and healthy eating a priority."   —Eve

"As a professional athlete my tendency was to overtrain. Harley has taught me to eat healthier, simplify my workouts, and maximize results."   —Rick Fox

"*5-Factor Fitness* offers a well-conceived, sensible, and useful plan that can be easily incorporated into an individual's lifestyle and that will yield positive health benefits."   —Roger Kelton, Ph.D.,
chair, School of Kinesiology and Health Science,
York University, Toronto

"While his charisma may inspire you, don't be fooled. Underneath lies a true pioneer in bringing science into the gym and the kitchen to help make fitness and nutrition a fundamental and easy part of our daily lives."   —David J. Klein, B.Sc. M.D.,
fellow, Critical Care Medicine, University of Toronto

"Personal trainer to the stars, Pasternak promises that in five weeks, working five days a week, eating five meals a day, and prepping for five minutes for five segments of five-minute workouts (got all those fives?) you, too, can look like Halle Berry in her catsuit."   —*Library Journal*

Factor Fitness

**THE DIET AND FITNESS SECRET
OF HOLLYWOOD'S A-LIST**

HARLEY PASTERNAK, M.Sc.
AND ETHAN BOLDT

A PERIGEE BOOK

THE BERKLEY PUBLISHING GROUP
Published by the Penguin Group
Penguin Group (USA) Inc.
375 Hudson Street, New York, New York 10014, USA
Penguin Group (Canada), 90 Eglinton Avenue East, Suite 700, Toronto, Ontario M4P 2Y3, Canada
(a division of Pearson Penguin Canada Inc.)
Penguin Books Ltd., 80 Strand, London WC2R 0RL, England
Penguin Group Ireland, 25 St. Stephen's Green, Dublin 2, Ireland (a division of Penguin Books Ltd.)
Penguin Group (Australia), 250 Camberwell Road, Camberwell, Victoria 3124, Australia
(a division of Pearson Australia Group Pty. Ltd.)
Penguin Books India Pvt. Ltd., 11 Community Centre, Panchsheel Park, New Delhi – 110 017, India
Penguin Group (NZ), cnr Airborne and Rosedale Roads, Albany, Auckland 1310, New Zealand
(a division of Pearson New Zealand Ltd.)
Penguin Books (South Africa) (Pty.) Ltd., 24 Sturdee Avenue, Rosebank, Johannesburg 2196, South Africa
Penguin Books Ltd., Registered Offices: 80 Strand, London WC2R 0RL, England

PRINTING HISTORY
G. P. Putnam's Sons hardcover edition / 2004
Perigee trade paperback edition / December 2005

PERIGEE is a registered trademark of Penguin Group (USA) Inc.
The "P" design is a trademark belonging to Penguin Group (USA) Inc.

The Library of Congress has cataloged the G. P. Putnam's Sons hardcover as follows

Pasternak, Harley.
5-Factor fitness : the diet and fitness secret of Hollywood's A-list / Harley Pasternak and Ethan Boldt.
p.   cm.
Includes index.
ISBN 0-399-15229-6
1. Physical fitness.   2. Exercise.   3. Reducing diets.
4. Celebrities—Health and hygiene.   I. Boldt, Ethan.   II. Title.
RA781.P296   2004   2004054795
613.7—dc22

PRINTED IN THE UNITED STATES OF AMERICA

10   9   8

Most Perigee Books are available at special quantity discounts for bulk purchases for sales promotions, premiums, fund-raising, or educational use. Special books, or book excerpts, can also be created to fit specific needs.

For details, write: Special Markets, The Berkley Publishing Group, 375 Hudson Street, New York, New York 10014.

TO MY MOM AND DAD,
TO WHOM I OWE EVERYTHING I HAVE
AND EVERYTHING I AM

ACKNOWLEDGMENTS

My literary agent Andrea Barzvi, for believing in me.

David Klein, for your friendship. You are a part of all my successes.

Halle Berry, because you were the spark that lit my fire to write this book.

Ethan Boldt, for helping me find the words, and Marc Haeringer, who fine-tuned them.

Pam Silverstein, for hooking me up.

Nuno, Stacey, Will, and Krishna, for holding down the fort.

My closest friends, Michael, Jamie, David, Jodi, Pierre, Anne, Steve, and James.

Don Carmody and Dr. Marvin Waxman, for the golden ticket.

Dr. Roger Kelton and Dr. Ira Jacobs, for teaching me how to teach.

My baby brothers, Jesse and Bobby: you may be taller, but I wrote a book.

Lucy and Viv: you are in my every thought.

CONTENTS

Harley Pasternak consistently looks at things differently, and exhibits a passion for what he does. The development of the 5-Factor Fitness program is a logical extension of his education and interest in health and fitness.

5-Factor Fitness captures the essence of a successful approach to physical fitness by applying Harley's creative version of the standard principles of balance, variety, stress modification, and minimal-time involvement to physical activity and eating. His program is innovative, applicable to all ages and adaptable for different lifestyles, yet safe and conservative in the best sense of the word. And he allows for the imperative "free choice" experiences, which are so often denied on other programs. His explanations and rationales of the various exercises and eating plans are simple and easy to understand and follow. His use of visual imagery for the exercises and building-a-house analogy for nutrition information make his work accessible to every reader, no matter what their level of experience or expertise.

5-Factor Fitness presents a well-conceived, sensible and useful plan that can be easily incorporated into an individual's lifestyle, and that will yield positive health benefits.

—Roger Kelton, Ph.D.

Chair, School of Kinesiology and Health Science,

York University, Toronto, Canada

Recently, I had a short layover in Chicago at O'Hare Airport, where I was grabbing a paper at the newsstand. Behind me in line were two women, one twenty-something and the other about forty-five. They were looking at a magazine and commenting on a photo of actress Halle Berry wearing a Catwoman suit. "How does she look like that? What is she doing?" "She's got to be starving herself." "Or she's working out three hours a day." I couldn't stop myself from turning around and assuring them, "No, she doesn't starve herself. She actually eats five meals and only works out for twenty-five minutes a day." Needless to say, they were incredulous. "Oh come on; where'd you hear that?" I admitted, "Because I train her."

On the plane, I thought about the women's reactions: they had peppered me with questions, such as, "What kind of meals? Guess it's easy for her, with a high-priced chef following her around." After I'd protested that the meals she eats are very simple and easy to prepare, I'd realized that I was talking to a rapt audience. It occurred to me then that I needed to get the word out about how attainable a great body is, for any of us.

So, what do Halle Berry, Benjamin Bratt, Orlando Bloom, pro basketball player Rick Fox, and rapper Eve all have in common, other than their celebrity? They use the 5-Factor method. They make regular top-10 appearances in those "Best Bodies in Hollywood" lists, and Halle was recently given the title of "Best Body in the World" by Reuters.

What if I told you they only worked out twenty-five minutes a day, five days a week? What if I told you that they ate five meals a day, with each meal requiring only five minutes to prepare? That's the 5-Factor.

You have in your hands a plan that works, and one that is very different from the methodologies you may have followed or heard about. The exercise part of 5-Factor takes very little time, yet is tremendously effective; and the eating portion is easy, satisfying, flexible, and won't alienate you from your family and friends.

The 5-Factor will work just as well for you as it has for my celebrity clients, and for me. Why? Because your physiology is no different from theirs, or my own. There really isn't a whole lot of variation in how the human body works, behaves, or responds to exercise. The benefits of 5-Factor are significant and apparent, no matter who you are.

Even though I won't be physically present with you, I will still guide you, every step of the way. Once you've read this book, you will know as much as any of my celebrity clients, and you will have the necessary tools to achieve the toned, lean, fit, and capable body of your dreams.

—*Harley Pasternak, M.Sc.*

PART

The Greatest Fitness-and-Food Program Ever Invented

1 · The Plan

I work with people who are motivated by the fact that their livelihoods hinge on how attractive they are. In fact, it's their calling card. I'm no different: I wouldn't be in very much demand as a fitness trainer if I didn't look extra-fit.

But while money and professional success are powerful motivators, so are many of the other good things that we want in life: love (a *big* motivator), approval, status, good health, boundless physical energy, strength, and the satisfaction of overcoming challenges.

Regardless of what is motivating you to change how you eat and exercise, I'm positive that you want to do it efficiently and painlessly. That's why I'm so excited to bring the 5-Factor to you. This is the simple plan that has kept Hollywood's A-List in shape for years.

I'm going to tell you right now exactly what you need to do over the course of the next five weeks to achieve the body you've always wanted. There are no hidden secrets. This is the same program that some of Hollywood's biggest stars use to stay in shape and look their best. Here is what you need to do:

- Eat five meals a day to boost your metabolism and reduce body fat

- Follow the five criteria for each meal—(1) low-fat quality protein (2) low- to moderate- glycemic index carbohydrate (3) fiber (4) healthy fat, and (5) sugar-free beverage—that will satisfy your appetite, deliver balanced nutrition, and keep your blood-sugar levels stable (preventing insulin spikes and subsequent fat storage). These criteria allow you to eat "normal" foods and "normal" amounts, yet also pave the way for significant fat loss and lean tissue preservation.

- Spend only five minutes preparing each meal, which requires only five easy-to-find ingredients.

- Work out twenty-five minutes, five days a week, for five weeks to get your body to lose fat, gain lean muscle, and increase energy in less time than any other program.

- Indulge in your weekly cheat day. That's right, one day a week indulge your cravings and eat the foods you love.

That's it. That is the simple program that has worked for countless people. No carbohydrate counting; no calorie counting; no measuring food; no long or complicated exercise routines; no major time commitment. This is what Hollywood insiders have known for years. Anyone can look like a celebrity; maybe you can't look like a specific celebrity, but, without question, *you* can look as though *you* are a star about to shoot a film, go on a record tour, or tape a music video.

You are reading this, so your interest is clearly piqued. But please don't leave it there—put it to use. The pleasure that you'll earn is a hundred times greater than the anxiety you may feel now, while wondering if *you* can pull it off. You can. You will.

2 · The 5-Factor Difference

Why You've Failed Before

Why does someone abandon a fitness or diet program? Simply because the severity of that program outweighs the benefits that it provides. The truth is, almost every weight-loss diet is doomed to failure. Usually it is severely restrictive in some respect: either by limiting you to so few calories, fat, or carbohydrate grams a day that going to a restaurant or eating at a friend's house becomes very difficult. Also, it requires extensive planning and diplomacy, and demands that you master complicated techniques and rules for meal preparation. Or, because you are miserably hungry the entire time, it leaves you *itching* for the diet to end, so you can resume your normal life.

Hence, strict diets are extremely tough to sustain week in and week out. The dropout rates of such diets are astonishingly high. What's more, the temptation to sabotage an onerous regimen is just too hard to resist. Many of my clients had tried numerous fitness-and-diet routines before mine; some had success with these routines, yet they often felt that the workouts were "hellish" and the diets "harsh." As a result, these plans were short-term fixes at best, but soon after the film or athletic season they had prepared for was over, they were back on the open road looking for something better. They found it with 5-Factor.

The 5-Factor is different—very different—from all of the programs you've tried before. The 5-Factor helps you instantly make big changes—losing fat, getting more lean muscle (and better body shape), and boosting your energy level—without turning your life upside down. In fact, it's easily incorporated into your busy life, because the workout takes only twenty-five minutes a day, five days a week. You don't have to go to a gym or see a trainer. And the meal plan is easy to follow. You'll be eating more often, while not carb or calorie counting.

Let's face it, we live in a land of excess in every respect but one: *time.* Have you ever been deterred from trying to gain control over your appearance and fitness by the thought of shoehorning a one- or two-hour workout into your already packed day? Has the thought that you might need to alter the way you and your family eat, perhaps by spending hours a week shopping for unfamiliar foods, plus devoting hours a day preparing complicated meals, stopped you from trying to get matters in hand? Have you hesitated to try making more nutritious, healthy meals, either because it will take tons of time and effort or because it might isolate you from others, by making you adopt an extreme eating style?

You won't encounter any of that with the 5-Factor. Here are the five reasons why other plans don't work and why the 5-Factor does:

1. They require too much time or equipment—5-Factor workouts only last twenty-five minutes and require only a bench and some dumbbells

2. They are boring—5-Factor workouts keep you engaged because you'll change the rep ranges, exercises, sequences, and muscle combinations continually

3. They are difficult to comprehend and follow—5-Factor exercises are simple and easy to master

4. They are built on outmoded principles, rather than on the latest scientific breakthroughs—the 5-Factor methodology I've used is backed by new, state-of-the-art research and findings

5. They require adherence to a dull, restrictive, or complicated diet—the 5-Factor diet you'll follow is one that is simple, balanced, and easily obtained, anywhere you are likely to go

Why the 5-Factor Will Work for You

I've noticed that when someone says to me, "I'm too busy to work out," or "I don't believe in all these diet plans; they all contradict one another," or "I'm not an athlete, nor do I want to be one, so there's no way I can sustain an exercise program," those declarations are actually questions in disguise.

Here are those disguised questions: "How much time will it take?" "How and what should I eat?" "Is working out going to be too hard for me? Can I really do it?"

Yes, you can.

"I don't have time to work out"—you can carve out twenty-five minutes in your day

"I don't want to join a gym"—you don't have to

"I don't have a place to exercise"—all you need is a bench and a set of dumbbells

"I don't know anything about exercise"—there are only three exercises per workout

"I can't eat in a deprived, freakish manner"—you won't be deprived (five meals per day), and you won't have to cut out any food groups

All the above concerns are those that I've heard from my own clients and in my years of training, studying, and talking to others. Probably you have at least a few of these yourself. I believe that these concerns, doubts, and fears stem from the fact that, until now, your relationship to exercise hasn't worked. Fortunately, you're in good hands, for the 5-Factor is the most revolutionary workout plan ever invented.

That's a bold statement that is backed up with scientific reasoning and straightforward facts. If you've never worked out before, then you got lucky your first time out. If you have trained before, you will appreciate this workout more than any other routine you've tried—for both its cutting-edge method as well as its extraordinary results.

When it comes to choosing a fitness plan, we all want the same thing: results, delivered to our bodies as quickly as possible. That's

FIVE BIG BENEFITS OF 5-FACTOR

What's the payoff? Plenty. There are five ways in which you will be rewarded:

1. Look better: the lean, perfectly balanced body will be yours
2. Perform better: whether in sports or in your daily life, your performance level is about to go up
3. Get more energy: the perfect level of training will energize you throughout your day
4. Earn better health: top-notch nutritional and training methods will make you healthier than ever
5. Enjoy better moods throughout the day: this type of intense, quick training spurs your body to release "feel-good" endorphins, while the eating plan moderates your blood-sugar level, which means that the dreaded "afternoon slump" is a thing of the past

called efficiency. We, however, also need efficacy: in other words, a program that is not only effective right out of the gate, but that will create positive changes with your body—less fat, more lean muscle, more energy—continually, for as long as you use the program.

What's the end result? How does losing at least 5 pounds of fat (and often more) while changing the shape of your body in five weeks sound? It may represent the final stage of where you want your body to be or, more likely, will be the first major step toward the body shape you've coveted for so long.

I'm confident that 5-Factor Fitness works because it's produced these exact results for my clients—clients who are actors and actresses who hire me before they begin filming a movie or go on a photo shoot. Five weeks is all it takes.

REAL RESULTS
Halle Berry • 36 • Actress

One of my favorite clients is Halle, who I first trained for a film called *Gothika*. She was known around the world for her beautiful body, to say nothing of her beautiful face. In her hometown of Los Angeles, she worked out hard and got results, yet some of her training had unduly stressed her joints. On top of some painful, nagging injuries, many sustained as a childhood gymnast, her physique was slightly unbalanced. While some of these problems were the result of improper training, many, in fact, emanated from *over*training.

After my third session with her, Halle had become so enamored with the 5-Factor that she asked me if I could come back with her to L.A. to train her for the movie *Catwoman*. I accepted.

Catwoman required her to be in tip-top physical condition. We wanted to develop better body balance, while becoming injury-free and sexier along the way. First, we redistributed some of her weight by getting more definition in her upper body. She had a flat stomach, but we made it stronger and leaner while keeping it sexy. Like many women, she had very powerful quadriceps but relatively weak and tight hamstrings; they were being overpowered and made her vulnerable to potential knee and lower-back injuries. So we worked to make the back of her legs and her butt more balanced as well as firmer. The most key exercises to her body improvement were the stiff-legged deadlifts for her hamstrings and the lunges for her butt.

Cardio was also a challenge because Halle, like many of us, hates to do it. Getting her to do long bouts of cardio was tough, but she knew she wanted to get leaner. So for a few weeks, we extended the fifth stage of the workout to thirty minutes. Doing that five times a week, plus the twenty minutes of stages 1 through 4, worked magic. Shooting began five weeks later and her body was in peak shape. At that point, we dropped the fifth stage back to five minutes.

With 5-Factor, Halle's body keeps progressing. Even though we almost never go beyond the twenty-five-minute workout, Halle keeps getting stronger and stronger—two full years after we began her 5-Factor journey.

PART

5-Factor Fitness

3 · The Science and Sense Behind 5-Factor Fitness

The 5-Factor Fitness portion asks for just twenty-five minutes five days a week, and each workout consists of only three exercises and ten minutes of cardio. For many of you, this is welcome news, though you may wonder in the back of your mind how it's possible to make substantial changes with such little time expenditure. Others may immediately declare that this workout can't be enough to meet their goals of fat reduction and lean muscle increases.

I'm here to ease and eradicate those fears. You will reap more gains from this routine than any previous one you've tried. Or if you've never really given any fitness program a try, you've chosen wisely. Why? It's simple. The 5-Factor optimizes efficiency, in terms of time *and* results.

The great results will come because of how the 5-Factor uses the mighty principles of variety and intensity. If you're worried that the program won't match your current fitness level (from out of shape to very fit), I've carefully designed two 5-Factor workouts:

levels I and II. Level I includes a one-week preparation phase for those new to exercise and/or those who have been sedentary for a long time.

> The 5-Factor is the only kind of workout that you can still do when you're sick, or feel a cold coming on. Research shows that short, intense workouts can assist immune-system function, while longer workouts may overtax the immune system.

How the 5-Factor Was Born

I first developed a passion for the subjects of fitness, health, and diet as a teen hockey player in Canada. In order to get stronger and more powerful on the ice, I began lifting weights (thanks, in part, to my mom, who first introduced me to the gym). Weight lifting became a lifelong habit when I witnessed the tremendous effect that it had on my body, psychology, and social life.

The ensuing years that I spent as an amateur bodybuilder, graduate student, and fitness trainer did nothing to diminish my enthusiasm. In fact, I became driven by the idea that there had to be an optimal way to train and eat, and that I was the guy who could and would find it.

I knew that the sheer volume of writings, videos, and magazine articles on these subjects testified to their universal appeal, but they remained rather mysterious to most people. I was consumed by the notion that there might be a key to solving the fitness-and-diet riddle, and that if I searched for it, I could find it.

My search continued during the first eight of my eleven years training others, until, four years ago, *I found it*. I discovered the elusive "holy grail" itself: an absolutely effective, safe, and efficient way to exercise and eat that was easily put into practice, with as minimal a time investment as possible.

What do I mean by "an absolutely effective, safe, and efficient way"? During my years of study and training, I'd found that there are dozens of possible ways to exercise and eat in order to lose fat and build lean muscle: strength training, intense cardiovascular activity, various sports, yoga, etc. The problem, of course, was that all of these methods required massive time commitments, with varying results. What I wanted was a program that would be extremely time-effective and easy to follow, and would deliver immediate results.

The Science

I began my quest for the perfect system in graduate school, when I was given the unique opportunity to conduct research with the Defense and Civil Institute of Environmental Medicine. I joined a group of scientists who were trying to examine the effects of nutritional supplements on physical performance, i.e., strength and endurance.

Fortunately, the pattern of the 5-Factor began to emerge early on. One particular study, assessing the effects of consumed nutritional supplements on muscular strength and endurance, used double-blind lab tests with exercises. After the subjects ingested capsules (real or placebo), they performed two exercises (a Smith-machine bench press and a 45-degree leg press), one immediately after the other without rest to exhaustion, three times. As the study progressed and with each weekly trial, the subjects grew stronger: in fact, their bodies became noticeably more muscular and fit. This was astounding, given that each exercise trial took only ten minutes. How could ten minutes of intense exercise once a week effect such a transformation?

Next, I examined the world-class Bulgarian powerlifting team, which produced Olympic champions yet trained only ten minutes at a time; their sports scientists discovered that higher levels of testosterone and growth hormone—the two principal hormones responsible for building muscle and burning fat—were secreted by the body during short, intense workouts rather than longer, more-tempered sessions. Next, I studied the training system developed by professional bodybuilder Mike Mentzer, the only competitor ever to earn a perfect score in a Mr. Universe competition—meaning that he had developed an absolutely perfectly balanced physique. He, too, believed that *intensity* was a far more significant exercise factor than duration in achieving body transformation.

I was able to refine my understanding of the concept of intensity by examining, next, the work of the Canadian endocrinologist Hans Selye, Ph.D., who devised, and then won a Nobel Prize for, a theory called the General Adaptation Syndrome (GAS). This theory led me to the discovery that *variation* was as essential as intensity—in the form of manipulating rep ranges and exercise sets (each set represents a group of reps) as well as weight loads—for the perfectly efficient workout. For example, if you keep exposing the same stress to the body, at some point we stop reacting to it. Do ten push-ups after not having done any exercise in months and you'll be sore the next day; start doing ten push-ups every day, however, and you not only won't be sore anymore, the push-ups will barely do you any good. Your body has *adapted*—and unlike the professional athletes who want their bodies to adapt to the rigors of their sport, you have a completely different goal in your training. You want to keep your body off-balance as much as possible.

When I viewed this idea in light of my own work—particularly the military field study—I realized that the enormous benefits of intensity and variation would best be realized if the program revolved around short, frequent workouts.

If you're a woman, the beautiful, shapely silhouette of the ballet dancer or the long muscular shape of the rower probably captures the kind of body you want. For the man, the powerful, athletic, and muscular sprinter's physique might fit the image you want.

What do these vocations have in common? They all utilize what is, in effect, an intense, very high-rep range. The ballet dancer springs across the floor dozens of times, the sprinter rockets down the track for forty strides, and the rower cranks the oars through the water hundreds of times. However, while you always have the option of taking up ballet, sprinting, or rowing, you'll have to spend hours practicing almost every day of the week—which is exactly what these folks do. Instead, with 5-Factor you will derive similar results from similarly intense high-rep ranges.

Varying the number of reps and sets constantly shocks the body, which includes your muscles (making you leaner and stronger), hormones (stimulating your metabolism), bones (protecting you against osteoporosis), and connective tissue (preventing repetitive stress and other injuries). Your "muscle potential" is simply not reached with short-rep ranges. You won't get the muscle shaping, calorie burn, and higher energy level—three attributes that all of us seek—in other programs that consistently keep the rep ranges under 15, and/or rarely vary the rep ranges from week to week.

Twenty-five minutes, five days per week, is all you need. I've designed the program to address the need for exercise variety. Our bodies are designed to strive toward reaching a "set point," where changes stop occurring—it's actually a survival mechanism. Consequently, during each week of the 5-Factor, you'll complete a different number of repetitions. Continue to demand new things from your muscles, and you will continue honing your physique.

The Five Training Variables of 5-Factor

One primary reason why the 5-Factor works so well is how it uses *variety*. As with everything, variety is the spice of life; it awakens you, whether it involves your route to work, the food you eat, or your sex life. The same goes with exercise, as your body responds more quickly and consistently when you use the variety principle.

In particular, for every week out of the five weeks, these five training variables (below) are shifted in order to ensure that your body never stops progressing.

1. Type of exercise (for strength training, cardiovascular, and core movements)

2. Repetitions

3. Sets

4. Resistance level

5. Rest periods

The Number "5"

The number "5" in 5-Factor was not chosen at random. It's actually integral to why this program works so well. After extensive research and further experimentation with myself and my client base, I found that five phases in a single workout represent the optimal training stimulus for beginner to advanced exercisers: a cardio warm-up, followed by two phases of strength training to develop lean muscle and boost your metabolism, one phase to work your crucial midsection, then ending with cardio to burn additional fat and cool your body down. The last cardio phase can be lengthened for the advanced exerciser. Because the workout is broken into five chunks of intense exercise that work your body differently, the 5-Factor workout is extremely doable—and you will be surprisingly refreshed for each workout.

For high-level fat burning, lean muscle gains, and metabolic boosting, five short workouts is optimal. More than five may push you into overtraining mode, straining your muscles, and fewer won't be enough to see significant results. Because your metabolism is elevated for up to forty-eight hours after a strength workout, it makes sense to create that benefit as often as possible. Additionally, I found that five-week cycles were sustainable and effective. Each participant lost at least 5 pounds of fat in those first five weeks (and beyond, if they were carrying excess fat) and gained more lean muscle.

Divide in Order to Conquer

The 5-Factor works your muscles in a revolutionary way. Most resistance-training programs split your body into different muscle groups to be trained and then designate these groups to different days of the week; others simply split the body in two, such as upper body and lower body; some even work the entire body in one workout. All of these have inherent problems—ranging from being ineffective, working only for a time, to overtraining—because they don't take three important matters into account.

First, the *time* you spend working a certain muscle should be proportional to the size of the muscle. Too often, I see men spend 75 percent of all their workout time on their chest and biceps, when these two muscles represent less than 20 percent of the body's muscle mass. Women are guilty, too. Many women spend most of their time working their butts and their front and inner thighs. In doing so they not only neglect the rest of their body, they also are creating dangerous muscle imbalances. The worst part of doing this is, they end up shortchanging their efforts to look like they've got slimmer thighs, because their underdeveloped shoulders, arms, and torsos contribute so much to that "thunder thigh" appearance.

Second, *balance* is more than merely an aesthetic concern: by training certain body parts too much and other parts not enough, you may be compromising your posture and putting yourself at risk for injury. By working opposing muscle groups equally—such as the hamstrings to the quadriceps, the rear shoulder to the chest/front shoulder—you will maintain a proper muscle balance and flexibility, thus reducing your susceptibility to injuries.

Third, when deciding what muscle groups to train together, it's imperative that you pay attention to the *psychological factor*. Our desire, or lack thereof, to work on a certain muscle group will directly affect the intensity with which we will train. Generally speaking, smaller muscles are much easier to train than larger muscles; as a result, many people dread training their legs. This huge muscle group represents more than half of all our muscle and causes our heart rate to soar and our muscles to burn. On the other hand, our arms and abs are much smaller muscles and do not create as much overall fatigue or high-calorie burn. The result, of course, is that many people look forward to training their arms and abs because they are easier to work. Less sweat, less pain. And when it comes to training the legs, for example, they either skip the workout or train them inadequately.

For this reason, I designed the 5-Factor to avoid the typical upper body/lower body split used by so many. I separate the work for the legs as well as for the main torso muscles. Because I don't expect you to get bogged down by exercise science, I want to highlight how significant this "separation" is: each of the five workouts is manageable for any level of ability or fitness.

The 5-Factor works the larger muscle groups (chest, quadriceps, back, and hamstrings) twice a week, while the smaller muscles (biceps, triceps, and shoulders) are worked once a week. The reason for that is simple: as a result of training our chest and back, we actually train our shoulder and arm muscles indirectly. For example, the chest-press exercise involves the shoulder and triceps muscles, while the back exercises involve the biceps and posterior shoulder. Because of their "part-time" job on the chest and back days, I actually consider working the shoulders and arms more than once per week to be overtraining.

Meanwhile, it's a very good idea to work the large muscles of the body twice a week and not just once. Why? First, because these muscles take up more mass than our smaller muscles and require more work. Second, these muscles literally "carry much of the load" when we move our bodies around during the week, so such a workout is very "functional." Third, to thoroughly train these large muscle groups, often two exercises that target different parts of the muscle group are necessary.

Putting It All Together (Intensity + Variety = 5-Factor)

In my experience as a trainer with my clients and as a scientist in a laboratory, the principles of intensity and variety were repeatedly found to be critical for producing the best kind of workout; moreover, these principles had to be instituted in a precise, well-designed program to be optimally effective as well as sustainable by anyone who wants to get in better shape.

By "intensity," I don't mean working out every muscle in your body every day. Doing so would neither be particularly effective nor be a program that you could stick with, year in and year out—or even for five weeks. Meanwhile, "variety" in the form of using multiple exercises in one workout, or doing something different every time you work out, is also not what I'm talking about. Both of these strategies may be effective but can also lead to overtraining or confusion.

Instead, with the 5-Factor, I've taken out all the guesswork for you by using intensity and variety in the most scientific yet simple way possible.

TEN MINUTES OF STRENGTH TRAINING A DAY BOOSTS YOUR BODY IN FIVE WAYS

The benefits of strength training are huge, and the 5-Factor yields them in only ten minutes per training day:

1. It revs up your metabolism and, as a result, helps you burn fat between workouts. Studies have shown that weight training for ten minutes puts your body in a state of recovery and boosts your metabolism for a full forty-eight hours after strength training versus only forty minutes if you do thirty minutes of cardio.

2. It prompts your body to release the right hormones to increase lean muscle tissue while burning fat stores.

3. It increases bone density. In fact, numerous studies show that osteoporosis can be prevented if you use a regular strength-training program.

4. It develops lean muscle. Recent clinical studies show that you can build muscle well into your nineties.

5. It builds balance. By using dumbbells in the 5-Factor program, you improve your balance, which will guard against injury and improve your coordination and dexterity in all your activities.

REAL RESULTS
Carmen Ingelstein • 74 • University Professor

One of the most amazing women I've had the good fortune to know, Carmen has published numerous books and spoken in more than forty countries around the world. Referred to me by her psychiatrist, she is a widow who suffered from depression and was also overweight and arthritic. She ate infrequently and barely exercised at all, falsely believing that she was too old.

The first time she came to my studio, she struggled to get up the stairs. Within days on the 5-Factor, however, she began to change dramatically. Once completely sedentary, she began riding her bike to my studio, would practically leap out of her chair, actually loved opportunities to carry heavy grocery bags, and went on to climb Mount Kilimanjaro and go on European bike trips. She also went off antidepressants, and her psychiatrist called to say she was in a better mental state than ever before. Out of all my clients, she is the one I am the most proud of.

4 · Getting Ready

**WHAT YOU NEED TO KNOW
BEFORE YOU WORK OUT**

If this represents your first real effort to exercise in quite some time, consider the 5-Factor the beginning of great changes that your body will make. First, by doing very high repetitions in week 1 and gradually decreasing the number of reps and increasing the weight over the following weeks, you are going to create a giant warm-up. You are priming your muscles, tendons, ligaments, and chemistry for more challenging workouts ahead.

If the 5-Factor is taking over from other workouts that you've recently used, I urge you to completely abandon those previous workouts. The 5-Factor is so comprehensive that carrying over any elements from others could result in overtraining.

Optimizing Your Workout

BEST TIME TO TRAIN

You've probably heard it before, but a great time to exercise is in the morning because the day doesn't get in the way. It sets the right tone for the day, and you don't have to find time or energy later in the day. Because the 5-Factor only takes twenty-five minutes, it's also simple to work out before your workday begins.

If the morning time does not suit you, then anchor your workout slot to some other daily routine, such as coming home from work (stopping by the gym, or hitting the weights the moment you walk in your front door) or over your lunch hour. (Both workouts, of course, presuppose that you've had a good, 5-Factor snack.)

The key point is this: *any time can work, as long as you have natural energy at that time.* Maybe nighttime is what fits you.

THE EQUIPMENT YOU NEED

Here it gets *very easy.* All you need are *dumbbells* and a *bench,* even if you belong to a fancy gym.

If you will work out at home, I can suggest many places to find dumbbells and a weight bench. You can go to your local sporting goods shop, including those that carry used equipment, all of which you can find through your Yellow Pages. You can also check the Internet and search under "gym equipment," "weight bench," and/or "dumbbells."

In terms of specific dumbbells, there are the all-in-one varieties, such as Powerblock, which offers two 5 to 50-pound dumbbells in which you use a pin to separate the weights. They cost several hundred dollars, however, so you may choose the more standard individual dumbbell, which can be everything from sand weights, rubber-coated, hexagonal, and on up. The cheapest option of all is buying two small dumbbell bars, made up of plastic or steel, to which you add weight plates (buying four 2.5-, 5-, and 10-pound plates each gives you 5-, 10-, 15-, 20-, 25-, 30-, and 35-pound dumbbells).

For most women, two individual dumbbells at 3, 5, 8, 10, and 12 pounds will get you started. Men should get 10-, 15-, 20-, 25-, and 30-pound dumbbells. If you realize that you need heavier weights, all you have to do is go out and buy some additional dumbbells; it can be a reward for your improving shape.

There is also a cardio component to the workout, of course. While you can go for a power walk or jog outside, you may prefer to work out in the privacy of your own home, especially if the outside environment isn't always conducive to exercise. Not too many places can accommodate jumping rope, so I'd recommend that you use a cardio machine (there are many designed for the home user), such as a treadmill, elliptical machine, stationary bike, stepper, rowing machine, etc. I find that treadmills encourage the most exercise retention simply because walking is the most natural cardio activity of all, so you don't mind doing it every day. However, because the cardio portion is minimally five minutes, you will be able to stick with almost any kind of cardio machine.

THE FIVE REASONS WHY DUMBBELLS ARE BETTER FOR YOU THAN EXERCISE MACHINES

1. Dumbbells, your own body resistance, and a bench thoroughly work your targeted muscle *plus* the "stabilizer" muscles that surround the targeted area. Machines, on the other hand, work neither the muscles you're trying to target nor the surrounding muscles adequately.

2. They "fit" anyone, regardless of size or age, whereas machines are designed to fit an arbitrary "average" body standard.

3. Dumbbells allow your joints and muscles to follow a motion that is natural for your body, while machines force your joints, ligaments, tendons, and muscles to follow a "prescribed" motion that not only doesn't work the surrounding muscle but also may be unnatural for you (potentially creating problems with certain joints, such as the knee, hip, shoulder, and elbow).

4. They allow you to train isolaterally, which means you can train each side of your body separately and thus avoid muscle imbalances. Machines worsen any strength discrepancy (such as imbalanced strength with the legs, chest, back, or shoulders) that you may have now (a common problem).

5. They give you a *minimum* of 250 exercises, but most gym machines will only give you 1, and the "home gyms" sold on TV might give you a maximum of 20; because they're machines, they are still inadequate exercises compared to dumbbell exercises.

YOUR WORKOUT SPACE

If you plan to work out at home, then create a place free of distractions. Maybe this place will be in your bedroom, the garage, or the basement; maybe it can be the start of your very own home gym.

MUSIC

Okay, it's not exactly fitness equipment, but it can boost anyone's workout. It can help raise your intensity level as well as make you look forward to working out. Whether it's the Beatles, Beyoncé, or Beethoven, choose music that gets your blood pumping. Usually, the more aggressive, upbeat, and fast tempo the beat, the more intense the workouts.

THE AMOUNT OF WEIGHT YOU LIFT

The amount of weight you use is determined by the number of repetitions required for each set. This means a lighter weight for higher repetitions and a heavier weight for fewer repetitions. Select a weight that allows you to *just barely* complete the prescribed number of repetitions while maintaining proper technique.

For example, if you are supposed to do twenty repetitions and you are unable to complete the set, or if you must use poor technique to reach twenty reps, lower the weight. If, on the other hand, you find that you were not fully challenged and could probably have done more than twenty reps, make it slightly heavier next set. After the first set of your first workout per body part, you will get a sense of what weights you should use for future sets and workouts.

Along those lines, I strongly recommend that you write down how much weight you use each workout. It will help inform your decision of how much weight to use the next week when you do fewer reps, and thus more weight (varying anywhere from 2.5 to 10 pounds more).

To give you a rough guideline for how much weight you should use in your first week of workouts in which you do very high reps, I suggest that you go as low as 3-pound dumbbells to no more than 20-pounders, even if you're as strong as an ox. You can always up the weight for the next set.

Pace yourself. Remember, you're doing either more reps or more sets or both than what you're used to. So don't jack up the weight for one ultimate set and have nothing left. Stay true to the rest times by using the appropriate weight loads.

PROPER EXERCISE FORM

It's very important to use good form not only to prevent any possible injury but also to get maximum benefit from an exercise. Follow the exercise descriptions and pictures very carefully.

If you're unfamiliar with a move, use very light weights in the beginning during the preparation phase so you get the motion down. At no point is it worth it to "cheat" and use poor form to complete a rep. For the 1 percent advantage you can gain, it's not worth it if you injure yourself. I always chuckle when people tell me they use the "cheating principle" with their biceps (using leverage or momentum to get in a few extra reps), for example. The only thing you're cheating by using momentum is your biceps themselves. Instead, simply take your muscle to failure the right way.

FINISH WHAT YOU START

Fatigue can often be mental as well as physical. The first couple of weeks may be especially challenging because you will feel general fatigue over your entire body rather than just your one muscle

REAL RESULTS
Steve • 45 • Producer

A busy Los Angeles film producer, Steve is always producing two or three films at the same time, which means he has little time to work out. In addition, years of running excessively and lifting weights improperly had damaged his knees and shoulders. He also had developed high blood pressure and was carrying too much fat, weighing about 235 pounds.

Using the twenty-five-minute 5-Factor workout only and following the 5-Factor food plan, he went down to 181 pounds while his strength went *up* over the course of five months. The training helped remove both his knee and rotator cuff problems. His blood pressure normalized. And perhaps most amazing of all, we were able to squeeze in every workout into his hectic day, principally because they last for only twenty-five minutes.

group. If your fatigue is mostly local, you can push through to the end of the set, if you're significantly motivated.

If you're huffing and puffing, stop halfway through the set, take a brief rest, and then resume the set to finish. Try to finish the recommended sets and reps, even if you have to lower the weights to almost nothing. Remind yourself that the strength-training portion is only ten minutes long. You can do it. (If you get dizzy or feel faint, however, please stop and wait until your doctor has given you clearance before resuming.)

In any case, be aware that there's a big difference between being sore and getting injured. If you've injured yourself and feel pain, then stop. If you feel light pain that goes away immediately when you stop exercising (this is much more common than injury, which is rare and almost entirely avoidable, thank goodness), then your muscles are simply tired.

5 · The Five-Week Plan

Weeks 1 and 2: The Foundation Stage

The first two weeks focus on extremely high repetitions, meaning you will use relatively light weights and few sets of each exercise. This is what I call the foundation stage. Like building a house, you will be laying the physiological foundations upon which you will build a leaner and healthier body. For those new to exercise or who are coming off a long layoff, I recommend beginning with the Preparation Week before going to week 1.

In my experience, high reps are tough for most people because their bodies aren't used to it. Men, in particular, may struggle with the high reps not because they can't do it, but because their egos get in the way and they insist on using heavier weights. To complete the high-rep sets and stick to the rest times, you have to use smaller dumbbells than in your average workout. Trust me when I tell you, *nobody* cares how much you are lifting, unless you are a professional athlete.

Due to the high number of repetitions per set, you will experience something called *general fatigue,* which is an overall fatigue rather than just referring to a single muscle group. The high repetitions will cause the heart rate to soar, leading to greater caloric expenditure. Unlike local fatigue, in which the muscle being worked fatigues and becomes the limiting factor of the workout, your body will tire before any one muscle or muscle group does.

Weeks 3 and 4: The Framing Stage

We have the foundation laid, including good technique and a solid fitness base gained from the first ten workouts. As a result, we can kick it up a notch. In short, we need to frame the house, so we lower the number of repetitions (and make the weights significantly heavier) from week 1 and also add an extra set of each exercise.

We will experience more *local fatigue,* which is specific fatigue of a certain muscle group. Unlike the foundation stage, our muscles will now fatigue before our bodies do. We may also experience a bit more muscle soreness after these workouts.

Week 5: The Finishing Stage

I liken this stage to drywalling and painting the house. With only ten repetitions per set, and with two more sets per workout than weeks 1 and 2, you use much more resistance than any of the previous weeks.

As you enter the finishing stage, you have already done high reps with low weight, moderate reps with moderate weight, and now you will further challenge your body with more weight and more sets.

6 · The 25-Minute Workout

The workout consists of five phases, each of which will take roughly five minutes to complete. The last phase, "cardio," can be extended past the five minutes if you choose.

Use this workout five days a week: Monday, Tuesday, Thursday, Friday, and Saturday. As you will see, this is a precisely planned workout, and each of these training days uses different strength training and "core" exercises, so follow exactly as written. Wednesday and Sunday are considered "off" days, but you can do additional cardio on one of those two days; this can be any form of cardiovascular exercise for 15 to 30 minutes in length or a recreational activity you may enjoy; i.e., swimming, tennis, or dance. I do recommend that you take at least one of these two days off to give your body better recovery.

If you're worried that this workout will be too challenging or not challenging enough, don't be. First, for phases 1 and 5 (the cardio phases), go at your own pace. Second, for phases 2 through 4, I've designed two different levels of workouts, including a "preparation week" for those who have little to no training experience.

Minutes 0:00–4:59

1: CARDIO WARM-UP (75 CAL)

Do some form of cardio exercise for five minutes, gradually increasing your speed and/or resistance level. The purpose of the initial cardio phase is threefold. First, the cardio warm-up acts to do just that: to warm your body up. Your heart will start pumping more blood to your body, which will help warm your muscles, tendons, ligaments, and joints. This will reduce your chance of injury significantly. In fact, a good warm-up is far more effective for injury prevention than stretching.

The intensity of your warm-up cardio session should be moderate to low at first. After a couple of minutes, increase the intensity slightly by either going faster or increasing the resistance level. This may require you to walk, cycle, or step faster. Or you can increase the incline on the treadmill or raise the resistance level on the stationary bike or elliptical machine.

The second purpose of your warm-up is to get your heart in the "fat-burning zone," also referred to as the "target heart rate zone," which is 65 to 85 percent of your maximum heart rate. Your warm-up should be challenging enough that by the end you are in your target heart rate zone.

To calculate your zone, use the following formula:

$$(220 - \text{age}) \times (0.65 \text{ to } 0.85) =$$
$$\text{target heart rate zone (in beats per minute)}$$

How do you find your heart rate when you exercise? No, you don't need a heart rate monitor, though they can be helpful, of course. Get a timepiece with a second hand or a digital clock, then use two fingers (your first and second) to gently press on either your carotid artery or your radial artery. Your carotid artery is located on both sides of the front of your neck, on either side of your windpipe; your radial artery is just above your palm in a straight line down from your thumb. Once you have found either one of these pulse sites, count how many beats there are in ten seconds. Multiply this number by six, and, voilà, you have your heart rate.

The chart below shows you where you want your heart rate to be when you do cardiovascular exercise:

AGE	FAT-BURNING ZONE (IN BEATS PER MINUTE)
20	130–170
25	127–166
30	124–162
35	120–157
40	117–153
45	114–149
50	111–145
55	107–140
60	104–136
65	101–132
70	98–128
75	94–123
80	91–119

By elevating your heart rate at the beginning of your workout, you will stay in the fat-burning mode throughout the strength and core component of the workout.

The third purpose of the cardio warm-up is to mentally prepare you for the rest of your workout. It is the "buffer" that separates the stresses of daily living from your stress-releasing, body-sculpting daily workout. Think of it as the appetizer before the main course.

As long as you do your cardio, I'm happy no matter what type you choose. However, I want to pass on some recommendations.

A few years ago, I attended a conference in San Francisco and opted to walk the fifteen blocks to the conference center from my hotel and back, several times a day. This was San Francisco, so this walk was very hilly and was more enjoyable and effective than any cardio I'd done before. Call it the "San Francisco Effect."

Then and now, I consider uphill-walking the greatest cardio exercise of all (either outside or at the highest incline on a treadmill). Not only does it take pressure off the knees, but it helps strengthen the back of the knee, a common weak spot for many people. It also tones the thigh, butt, hamstring, and calf areas better than most cardio exercises because of the inclined walking surface. And because it's "walking," it *seems* easier to do than many other cardio options.

Two other top cardio exercises are stair-walking (with real stairs in a building, outside at a stadium, or on a step machine) and jumping rope, for similar reasons.

Because it's the most challenging cardio exercise of all, jumping rope burns more calories per minute than most other activities, and is low-impact compared to the second-most calorie-burning activity, running.

Other good cardio options include the elliptical machine, biking (stationary, recumbent, or mobile), rowing machine, and cross-country-skiing (not an easy option, but a great one if you have it). Meanwhile, many kinds of sports can deliver an excellent cardio workout, especially basketball, soccer, and tennis.

Doing different kinds of cardio, aka cross training, during one session or each time you work out, is an oft-recommended technique to raise the calorie burn and get in shape more quickly, but I find that it delivers these advantages simply because it allows you to exercise harder and for a longer duration than with your "pet" cardio activities.

Rather, the best reasons why you might use cross training are to avoid repetitive stress injuries and to keep things exciting for your brain (as well as your body). The hill-walker may want to get on a bike, or the rower use the elliptical machine. Or it may be as simple as changing the route that you take on your shoes, bike, or Roller Blades.

One type of cardio conspicuously absent from the above list is running. I discourage it for several reasons. The impact of running is two-and-a-half times your body weight for every stride and can lead to injuries to your feet, ankles, shins, knees, hips, and back. For women, running may also cause the breasts to permanently sag, even if you use the best sports bra available. The suspensatory ligaments that hold the breasts up stretch a little bit each time your breasts bounce up and down when you run. Women also have wider hips relative to men, and this causes several problems, including an increased hip-to-knee ratio that makes women more vulnerable to knee injuries.

If you love the running action and the huge number of calories it burns, consider *sprinting*. It's actually much better for you than jogging because all your force is propelled forward rather than up and down. Whether on a treadmill or on grass, a set of ten sprints is a fast, effective workout for people who are already in moderate shape and aren't carrying too much fat on their frame.

If you consider yourself to be out of shape, begin with the most natural movement of all: the walk. Work to increase your walking speed to over four miles per hour on level ground and eventually add an incline, at which point your walking speed will naturally decrease because of the added intensity.

Minutes 5:00–14:59

2 AND 3: STRENGTH TRAINING

For these two phases in each workout, there are two exercises, each working a different muscle group. Do them in the order suggested, and do the second exercise immediately after completing the set of the first exercise, which is called a *superset*. Then rest the suggested length before beginning the next superset. Follow this sequence for the recommended number of supersets.

In addition, if you go just under or just over the recommended number of reps, that's fine as long as you continue until you can physically no longer complete a rep with good exercise form. In order to get the maximum benefit of each exercise and stay injury-free, use good form by following the exercise descriptions and pictures carefully.

Note that each week as the total number of reps go down, your rest time also goes down but the weight you lift should go up. This will assure that the intensity level remains consistent.

Before I list all the exercise specifics, please heed this advice: the 5-Factor is a program I not only want you to try but also to complete. So stick to the rest times and rep ranges as well as you can, but if occasionally you need the extra rest or can't finish out a set, don't punish yourself by quitting. Take a breather and come back stronger. Remind yourself: only two exercises. Only ten minutes. I can do it!

During minutes 5:00 through 14:59, your week looks like this:

DAY	1 · MON	2 · TUES	3 · WED	4 · THURS	5 · FRI	6 · SAT	7 · SUN
Muscles	Chest Quads	Back Hams	OFF	Chest Quads	Shoulders Back	Biceps Triceps	OFF

LEVEL I STRENGTH TRAINING

Recommended for relative newcomers to strength training

PREPARATION WEEK:

2 sets of 15 reps of each exercise, with 90 seconds rest after doing the superset of 2 exercises back-to-back

WEEK 1:

2 sets of 25 reps of each exercise, with 80 seconds rest after each superset

WEEK 2:

3 sets of 20 reps of each exercise, with 70 seconds rest after each superset

WEEK 3:

3 sets of 15 reps of each exercise, with 60 seconds rest after each superset

WEEK 4:

4 sets of 12 reps of each exercise, with 50 seconds rest after each superset

WEEK 5:

4 sets of 10 reps of each exercise, with 40 seconds rest after each superset

LEVEL II STRENGTH TRAINING

For advanced exercisers, or after you've successfully
completed five weeks of Level I

WEEK 1:

3 sets of 30 reps, with 90 seconds rest after each superset

WEEK 2:

3 sets of 25 reps, with 70 seconds rest after each superset

WEEK 3:

4 sets of 20 reps, with 50 seconds rest after each superset

WEEK 4:

4 sets of 15 reps, with 40 seconds rest after each superset

WEEK 5:

5 sets of 10 reps, with 30 seconds rest after each superset

· DAY 1: MONDAY ·

CHEST: DUMBBELL CHEST FLY

Lie flat on the bench with your feet together tucked next to your butt. Hold the dumbbells with your arms extended toward the ceiling, palms facing each other and elbows slightly bent. *Inhale* as you bring the dumbbells away from each other toward the ground and open your chest. When you feel a comfortable stretch in the outer chest muscles, *exhale* and bring the dumbbells back toward each other. *Mental cue: imagine you're hugging a barrel.*

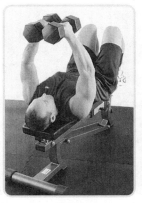

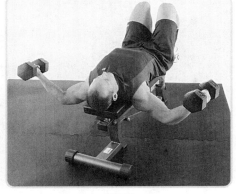

START   FINISH

QUADRICEPS: DUMBBELL TAP SQUAT

Sit on the end of the bench, holding a dumbbell in each hand, with your arms extended down toward the ground, palms facing each other, head up, shoulders back, and feet shoulder-width apart. *Exhale* as you stand up, then *inhale* as you sit down. As soon as your butt taps the bench, stand back up. *Mental cue: treat the bench as a chair behind you, so you sit down by moving your hips backward and down rather than just down.*

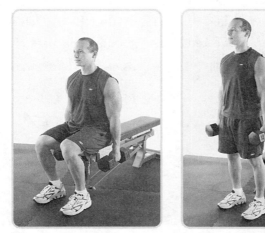

START   FINISH

· DAY 2: TUESDAY ·

BACK: SINGLE-ARM DUMBBELL ROW

Start off on the right side of the bench. Place your left knee, left lower leg, and left hand on the bench. Place the right leg out and back from the bench, with your right foot firmly planted on the ground, which creates a stable base of support. With your spine parallel to the floor, hold the dumbbell in your right hand with your right arm extending to the floor. With your palm facing the bench, *exhale* as you draw your elbow up along your ribs as high as you can. *Inhale* as you return the dumbbell back toward the starting position. Switch sides after completing a set. *Mental cue: elbow to ceiling and punch the ground.*

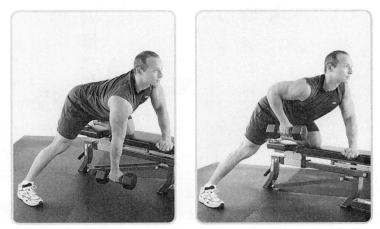

START   FINISH

HAMSTRINGS: DUMBBELL STIFF-LEGGED DEADLIFT

Place your feet shoulder-width apart and slightly bend your knees. Hold a dumbbell in each hand, with each dumbbell placed between the front and side of each thigh. With your head up and shoulders back, slide your hips backward as you *inhale*. Keeping your weight on your heel and an arch in your lower back, allow the dumbbells to slide down your thighs. When you can no longer push your hips backward, *exhale* and begin to slide your hips forward, and your upper body and the dumbbells will follow. *Mental cue: hit the wall behind you with your butt.*

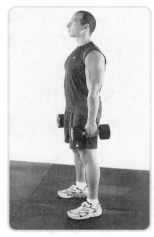

START

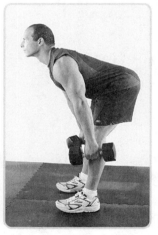

FINISH

· DAY 4: THURSDAY ·

CHEST: DUMBBELL CHEST PRESS

Lie flat on the bench with your feet up on the bench. Hold the dumbbells with your arms extended toward the ceiling, with both palms facing forward. *Inhale* as you gradually bring the dumbbells away from each other by hinging at the elbows and dropping them toward the floor. Once you feel a stretch in the chest and your hands are almost at chest level, *exhale* as you push the dumbbells back up toward the ceiling and each other. *Mental cue: imagine that you are balancing a glass of water on a tray in each hand, which will ensure correct elbow/arm angle and pace.*

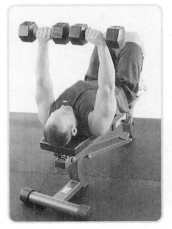

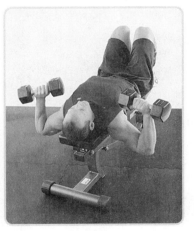

START   FINISH

QUADRICEPS/HAMSTRINGS:
DUMBBELL LUNGE

Stand with your feet shoulder-width apart and hold the dumbbells at arms' length, with your palms facing each other. (If you choose to go without dumbbells for this move, then place your hands on your hips.) With your shoulders back and head up, *inhale* as you take a large step forward. Lower your body so that you create a series of 90-degree angles (i.e., at the leading left leg, left ankle, left knee, left hip, as well as the back right knee and right ankle). As your back right knee nears the ground, *exhale* as you drive back with the muscles of your front leg to the starting position. Alternate after each rep. *Mental cue: imagine being knighted or proposing marriage!*

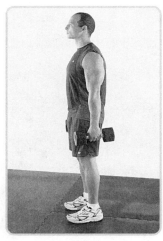

START

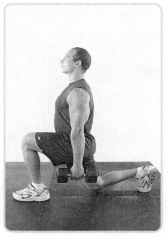

FINISH

· DAY 5: FRIDAY ·

SHOULDERS:
SEATED DB SHOULDER PRESS

Sit upright on the end of the bench with a dumbbell in each hand, palms facing forward and dumbbells on either side of your head. *Exhale* as you drive the dumbbells up toward the ceiling and each other, then *inhale* as you slowly return to the starting position. *Mental cue: reach for the ceiling as if you're cheering on your favorite team.*

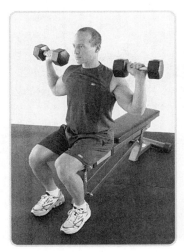

START

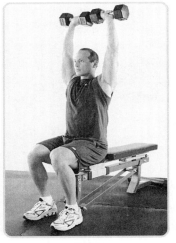

FINISH

BACK: DB PULLOVER

Lie flat on the bench with your feet up on the bench. Hold a single dumbbell directly above your chest by cupping the upper head of the dumbbell with both palms overlapping. With your elbows slightly bent, *inhale* as you gradually reach back behind your head and bring the dumbbell toward the ground until you feel a stretch in your lat muscles (outer back). *Exhale* as you return to the starting position. *Mental cue: imagine throwing a ball in slow motion into the sky with your arms only slightly bent.*

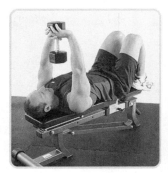 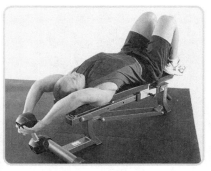

START   FINISH

· DAY 6: SATURDAY ·

BICEPS: DB HAMMER BICEPS CURL

Sit on the end of the bench and grasp a dumbbell in each hand with your arms extended downward and your palms facing each other. With your upper arms welded to your rib cage, *exhale* as you hinge at the elbows and bring each head of the dumbbell up toward your shoulders, then *inhale* as you return to the starting position. Do both arms at the same time and keep the palms facing each other throughout the whole set. *Mental cue: imagine raising a hammer up in each hand and then letting it drop down.*

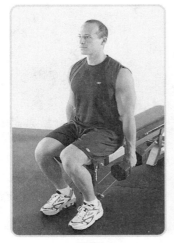
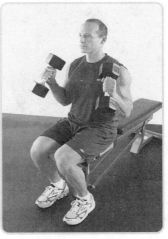

START   FINISH

TRICEPS: DB LYING TRICEPS EXTENSION

Lie flat on the bench with your feet up on the bench, tucked next to your butt. Hold a dumbbell in each hand, with your arms extended toward the ceiling and palms facing each other. *Inhale* as you hinge at the elbows and bring the dumbbells simultaneously down past your ears and toward your shoulders, then *exhale* as you press the dumbbells back to the starting position. Keep your upper arms still throughout the movement. *Mental cue: imagine hammering a nail into the ceiling with both arms.*

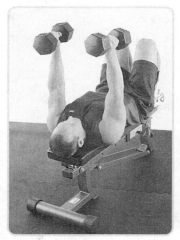 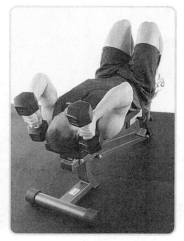

START   FINISH

Minutes 15:00–19:59

4: CORE EXERCISES

You want to develop a six pack? Tighten your tummy? Build a strong back? You want to get rid of that pooch? Those love handles? The 5-Factor will get it done because it works your entire midsection (i.e., the *obliques, transverse abdominis,* and *rectus abdominis*), whereas most programs only train the *rectus abdominus.*

But why does the core matter, for those of us who aren't going to be photographed on the beach anytime soon? Because the core is the most important muscle group, since it provides the foundation for all movements—everything from normal daily movements like getting out of bed or picking the paper up off the driveway to almost any physical activity that involves throwing or swinging, i.e., boxing, golf, tennis, or softball. It also serves to hold in our organs and stand upright with good posture. The upper body meets the lower body in the core, in which we are able to move in three planes. We can bend forward and backward, go side to side, and twist around. It's also why we work a different section of it every training day.

One part of the core that you don't want to overwork is the *erector spinae* (the lower back muscles), because it's activated all day long carrying you around and holding you up, whether you sit or stand. What's more, the lower back is particularly prone to injury—it's better to shore up the surrounding muscles, thereby reducing your likelihood of injury.

As a result, 5-Factor separates out your core into three sections—*rectus abdominis, transverse abdominis,* and *obliques*—and works them one to two times per week. Fitness magazines love to tell you about this great "core move," but there is no such thing as a complete core exercise. Most commonly, the transverse abdominis (the "corset") and the obliques (the "side abs") are ignored, while the rectus abdominis (the "washboard") is overtrained.

The diagram below illustrates the three key muscles of the mid-section.

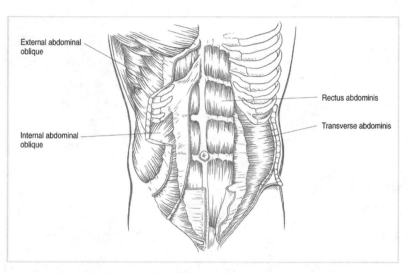

SOURCE: *ACE PERSONAL TRAINER MANUAL, 3RD EDITION* (2003). REPRINTED WITH PERMISSION FROM THE AMERICAN COUNCIL ON EXERCISE (WWW.ACEFITNESS.ORG).

The first, and certainly best known, is the rectus abdominis (RA)—often referred to as "the abs"—which runs from the bottom of your rib cage to the top of your pelvis. Located front and center, it acts primarily to flex the spine (bringing the rib cage closer to the pelvis, or chest to belly button, and vice versa); any time the belly button and the sternum move toward each other (otherwise referred to as a "crunch"), the RA is working. Because this muscle creates movement in our upper and lower body, we often split up into upper and lower RA.

The oblique muscles (internal and external), which lie under the skin and fat of the dreaded "love handle" region, are located on the sides of the core. They allow us to bend sideways. The external obliques originate along the lateral (side) portion of the ribs and attach to the crest of the pelvis. Conversely, the internal obliques originate along the crest of the pelvis and fan out to insert to the pubic bones and the ribs. The obliques act together to help in lateral flexion and torsion (twisting), yet are mostly ignored in typical ab training.

The third, and undoubtedly most neglected, core muscle is the transverse abdominis (TA). This corsetlike muscle wraps around your core and holds your organs in, and is really *the key to having a smaller midsection.* You use your TA muscle any time you twist around your spine, and it's essential for trunk stability.

Most people tend to focus only on the parts of their bodies they can see, so naturally the RA gets overworked. Further, people wrongfully assume that strong core muscles in the front will give them a lean tummy. This is not the case. As you will find out, diet and cardio plus comprehensive ab training are the way to get a defined, lean midsection.

Each of the first four training days focuses on four different regions of your midsection, or "core"; the fifth day will combine two of the regions. You will perform one abdominal exercise per day.

DAY	1 · MON	2 · TUES	3 · WED	4 · THURS	5 · FRI	6 · SAT	7 · SUN
Core Muscles	Upper Rectus Abdominis	Lateral Obliques	OFF	Lower Rectus Abdominis	Transverse Abdominis	Upper/ Lower Rectus Abdominis	OFF

As in stages 2 and 3, I've developed two different levels. Level I is appropriate for beginning to intermediate exercisers, while level II fits more advanced exercisers.

You will do the inverse number of sets and reps as you do with the strength training. As a result, you will do more sets with fewer reps and less rest in the first couple of weeks, and do fewer sets with more reps with longer rest by the end. Choose the level that corresponds to your strength training (stages 2 and 3).

Core Exercise

LEVEL I

PREPARATION WEEK:

3 sets of 10 reps, with 30 seconds of rest after each set

WEEK 1:

4 sets of 10 reps, with 15 seconds of rest after each set

WEEK 2:

4 sets of 12 reps, with 20 seconds of rest after each set

WEEK 3:

3 sets of 15 reps, with 25 seconds of rest after each set

WEEK 4:

3 sets of 20 reps, with 30 seconds of rest after each set

WEEK 5:

2 sets of 25 reps, with 35 seconds of rest after each set

LEVEL II

WEEK 1:

  5 sets of 10 reps, with 10 seconds of rest after each set

WEEK 2:

  4 sets of 15 reps, with 15 seconds of rest after each set

WEEK 3:

  4 sets of 20 reps, with 20 seconds of rest after each set

WEEK 4:

  3 sets of 25 reps, with 25 seconds of rest after each set

WEEK 5:

  3 sets of 30 reps, with 30 seconds of rest after each set

· DAY 1: MONDAY ·

UPPER-BODY CRUNCH

Lie on your back on a padded surface with your knees bent and your feet flat on the floor. With your hands beside your head, tuck your chin into your chest. *Exhale* as you bring your rib cage toward your pelvis, then *inhale* as you lie back and return to starting position. Keep your lower back on the ground at all times. *Mental cue: shorten the distance between your sternum and belly button on the way up, and lengthen it on the way down.*

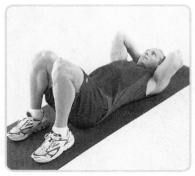
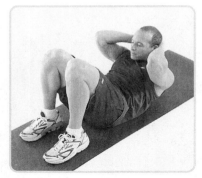

START   FINISH

· DAY 2: TUESDAY ·

DUMBBELL LATERAL FLEXION/EXTENSION

Stand with your feet slightly wider than shoulder-width apart. Hold a dumbbell in your left hand next to your left thigh. With both palms facing each other, slowly slide the dumbbell down your leg until you reach the bottom of the range of motion. Next, draw the dumbbell back up your thigh until the top of the range of motion. Keep your hips still throughout the movement. Upon completing the set, switch the dumbbell to other side. *Mental cue: imagine pivoting around your belly button.*

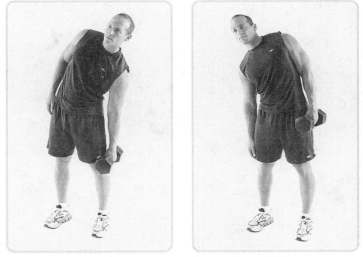

START **FINISH**

LOWER-BODY CRUNCH

Lie on your back with your feet off the ground, heels near your butt, and toes pointing down. Place your palms flat on the ground next to your hips and keep your hamstrings contracted and knees bent throughout the movement. *Exhale* as you roll your thighs and hips toward your chest, then *inhale* as you return three-quarters of the way back. *Mental cue: bring your belly button in toward your sternum.*

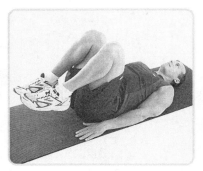

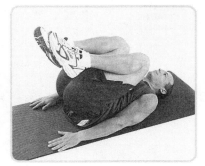

START
FINISH

· DAY 5: FRIDAY ·

UPPER-BODY TWIST

Sit on the mat with your knees slightly bent and toes facing up. Lean back slightly with your upper body and keep your head and hips still. *Exhale* as you reach across your body with your right hand and turn your chest toward the left wall, then *inhale* as you return to center. Then *exhale* again as you reach with your left hand and turn your chest toward the right wall. Go to both sides for each rep. *Mental cue: imagine reaching out and grabbing something on either wall, immediately sideways from you.*

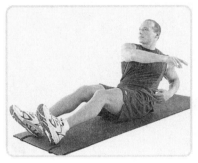

START

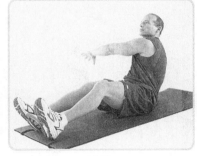

FINISH

· DAY 6: SATURDAY ·

DOUBLE-CRUNCH

This move is a combination of the upper- and lower-body crunches. Lie on a mat with your knees bent, feet beside your butt, toes pointed down, and hands behind your head. *Exhale* as you simultaneously crunch your lower and upper body at once, or roll your thighs and pelvis toward your chest while rolling your upper body toward your thighs, then *inhale* as you return to the starting position. *Mental cue: fold your body up like a clam by bringing your sternum and belly button toward each other.*

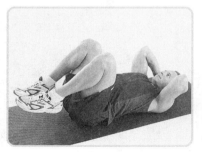

START

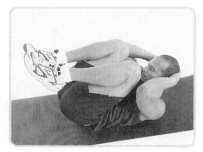

FINISH

Minutes 20–24:59 (or more)

5: CARDIO

Perhaps unlike the first five minutes, your body will welcome the natural, steady cardio rhythm at this point in the workout. Put in five good minutes of cardio, or go longer (up to thirty minutes) if you feel like it.

The goal of this final workout phase is twofold. First, we are actually trying to get your heart rate back up into the target heart rate zone. While it's important to increase the level of difficulty (speed and/or incline) as you become more fit and to vary the kind of cardio you do for a different mental stimulus (and to avoid repetitive stress injuries, especially if you're a runner), arriving at the fat-burn zone is most important. This contributes to the overall fat-burning effect of the workout. In fact, by this point in the workout (the twentieth minute), your body is accessing your fat stores for energy, and this "access" will continue at the same rate until you stop (the twenty-fifth minute or all the way to the forty-ninth minute). I don't recommend that you go over thirty minutes of extra cardio because that means you're less likely to go again tomorrow. Remember, you're working out almost every day. Getting in shape is a marathon, not a sprint.

Second, we finish the workout with cardio to enhance recovery and to "cool down" the body. Acute recovery from the resistance training occurs immediately. During the cardio phase lactic acid and carbon dioxide (both toxins) are flushed from the body following their production and accumulation, and nutrient-rich blood is produced to help your muscles recover and rebuild. The cooldown also fully loosens otherwise tight muscles and decreases something called delayed onset muscle soreness (DOMS). DOMS is the muscle pain you feel one to three days after a workout; those of you who have experienced DOMS before know exactly what I am talking about. A cardio cooldown will decrease the frequency and severity of DOMS.

Before you take off, I want you to understand OBLA. OBLA stands for onset of blood lactic acid, which occurs just before you hit fatigue; once you start accumulating OBLA, your muscles start shutting down. But everybody has different levels; exercise just below your OBLA, and you can go on forever. Let's say your OBLA level is 8.5: stay at 8.4 and you can go much faster, but increase it to 8.6 and you'll burn out in seven minutes. As a result, if you intend to go for longer than the five-minute cardio period, experiment to find that level that challenges your body yet doesn't overly fatigue it too early.

5-Factor Workout Charts

The charts for level I and level II follow, which I recommend that you photocopy for your workouts. On the photocopy, check off each completed workout and, for future reference as well as a record of your progress, write in the amount of weight you use for the strength-training exercises.

To lose additional fat, bring physical activities into other parts of your day. The reality is that with cars, TVs, and desk jobs, many of us simply aren't very active. But the workout shouldn't be the only time your body moves all day long. As I mentioned above, many of my clients from the entertainment industry only do the minimum of cardio (ten minutes per day), but they also have very active occupations and are often on their feet for much of the day.

I'm not saying that you should throw away your TV and start biking to work, but there are many small things that you can do to make your day more active. Over time, these moves will add up to a hundred or so more calories per day, which means an added weight loss of a pound or so a month. That's significant, especially over time.

Here are some suggestions: take the stairs instead of the elevator; get off the subway one stop earlier when going to work and coming home; in the parking lot, choose the spot farthest away from the store; shop in a pedestrian-friendly shopping area; occasionally walk to the place where you have lunch or dinner that day; plan leisure activities that involve movement (the mall, museums, walking tours, hikes, out-door games, amusement parks, etc.).

Day		Day 1	Day 2	Day 3
Phase/Time		Monday	Tuesday	Wednesday
Phase 1: Cardio 5 minutes		Cardio Warm-up	Cardio Warm-up	Cardio Optional
Phases 2 and 3: Strength Training 10 minutes		DB Chest Fly —— DB Tap Squat	Single-arm DB Row —— DB Stiff-legged Deadlift	Off
	Prep Week	15 reps each exercise	15 reps each exercise	
		Rest: 90 seconds	Rest: 90 seconds	
		Repeat	Repeat	
	Week 1	25 reps each exercise	25 reps each exercise	
		Rest: 80 seconds	Rest: 80 seconds	
		Repeat	Repeat	
	Week 2	20 reps each exercise	20 reps each exercise	
		Rest: 70 seconds	Rest: 70 seconds	
		Repeat 2 more times	Repeat 2 more times	
	Week 3	15 reps each exercise	15 reps each exercise	
		Rest: 60 seconds	Rest: 60 seconds	
		Repeat 2 more times	Repeat 2 more times	
	Week 4	12 reps each exercise	12 reps each exercise	
		Rest: 50 seconds	Rest: 50 seconds	
		Repeat 3 more times	Repeat 3 more times	
	Week 5	10 reps each exercise	10 reps each exercise	
		Rest: 40 seconds	Rest: 40 seconds	
		Repeat 3 more times	Repeat 3 more times	

WORKOUT: LEVEL I

Day 4 Thursday	Day 5 Friday	Day 6 Saturday	Day Sunday
Cardio Warm-up	Cardio Warm-up	Cardio Warm-up	Off
DB Chest Press —— DB Lunge	Seated DB Shoulder Press —— DB Pullover	DB Hammer Biceps Curl —— DB Lying Triceps Extension	Off
15 reps each exercise	15 reps each exercise	15 reps each exercise	
Rest: 90 seconds	Rest: 90 seconds	Rest: 90 seconds	
Repeat	Repeat	Repeat	
25 reps each exercise	25 reps each exercise	25 reps each exercise	
Rest: 80 seconds	Rest: 80 seconds	Rest: 80 seconds	
Repeat	Repeat	Repeat	
20 reps each exercise	20 reps each exercise	20 reps each exercise	
Rest: 70 seconds	Rest: 70 seconds	Rest: 70 seconds	
Repeat 2 more times	Repeat 2 more times	Repeat 2 more times	
15 reps each exercise	15 reps each exercise	15 reps each exercise	
Rest: 60 seconds	Rest: 60 seconds	Rest: 60 seconds	
Repeat 2 more times	Repeat 2 more times	Repeat 2 more times	
12 reps each exercise	12 reps each exercise	12 reps each exercise	
Rest: 50 seconds	Rest: 50 seconds	Rest: 50 seconds	
Repeat 3 more times	Repeat 3 more times	Repeat 3 more times	
10 reps each exercise	10 reps each exercise	10 reps each exercise	
Rest: 40 seconds	Rest: 40 seconds	Rest: 40 seconds	
Repeat 3 more times	Repeat 3 more times	Repeat 3 more times	

(Continued next page)

5-Factor Fitness

Day	Day 1	Day 2	Day 3
Phase/Time	Monday	Tuesday	Wednesday
Phase 4: Core 5 minutes	Upper-body Crunch	DB Lateral Flex/Extension	Off
Prep Week	10 reps each exercise	10 reps each exercise	
	Rest: 30 seconds	Rest: 30 seconds	
	Repeat 2 more times	Repeat 2 more times	
Week 1	10 reps each exercise	10 reps each exercise	
	Rest: 15 seconds	Rest: 15 seconds	
	Repeat 3 more times	Repeat 3 more times	
Week 2	12 reps each exercise	12 reps each exercise	
	Rest: 20 seconds	Rest: 20 seconds	
	Repeat 3 more times	Repeat 3 more times	
Week 3	15 reps each exercise	15 reps each exercise	
	Rest: 25 seconds	Rest: 25 seconds	
	Repeat 2 more times	Repeat 2 more times	
Week 4	20 reps each exercise	20 reps each exercise	
	Rest: 30 seconds	Rest: 30 seconds	
	Repeat 2 more times	Repeat 2 more times	
Week 5	25 reps each exercise	25 reps each exercise	
	Rest: 35 seconds	Rest: 35 seconds	
	Repeat 2 more times	Repeat 2 more times	
Phase 5: Cardio 5 minutes (or more optional)	Cardio	Cardio	Cardio Optional

Legend: DB = Dumbbell

WORKOUT: LEVEL I (CONTINUED)

Day 4 Thursday	Day 5 Friday	Day 6 Saturday	Day Sunday
Lower-body Crunch	Upper-body Twists	Double-Crunch	Off
10 reps each exercise	10 reps each exercise	10 reps each exercise	
Rest: 30 seconds	Rest: 30 seconds	Rest: 30 seconds	
Repeat 2 more times	Repeat 2 more times	Repeat 2 more times	
10 reps each exercise	10 reps each exercise	10 reps each exercise	
Rest: 15 seconds	Rest: 15 seconds	Rest: 15 seconds	
Repeat 3 more times	Repeat 3 more times	Repeat 3 more times	
12 reps each exercise	12 reps each exercise	12 reps each exercise	
Rest: 20 seconds	Rest: 20 seconds	Rest: 20 seconds	
Repeat 3 more times	Repeat 3 more times	Repeat 3 more times	
15 reps each exercise	15 reps each exercise	15 reps each exercise	
Rest: 25 seconds	Rest: 25 seconds	Rest: 25 seconds	
Repeat 2 more times	Repeat 2 more times	Repeat 2 more times	
20 reps each exercise	20 reps each exercise	20 reps each exercise	
Rest: 30 seconds	Rest: 30 seconds	Rest: 30 seconds	
Repeat 2 more times	Repeat 2 more times	Repeat 2 more times	
25 reps each exercise	25 reps each exercise	25 reps each exercise	
Rest: 35 seconds	Rest: 35 seconds	Rest: 35 seconds	
Repeat 2 more times	Repeat 2 more times	Repeat 2 more times	
Cardio	Cardio	Cardio	Off

5-FACTOR FITNESS

Day	Day 1	Day 2	Day 3
Phase/Time	Monday	Tuesday	Wednesday
Phase 1: Cardio 5 minutes	Cardio Warm-up	Cardio Warm-up	Cardio Optional
Phases 2 and 3: Strength Training 10 minutes	DB Chest Fly ——— DB Tap Squat	Single-arm DB Row ——— DB Stiff-legged Deadlift	Off
Week 1	30 reps each exercise	30 reps each exercise	
Week 1	Rest: 90 seconds	Rest: 90 seconds	
Week 1	Repeat 2 more times	Repeat 2 more times	
Week 2	25 reps each exercise	25 reps each exercise	
Week 2	Rest: 70 seconds	Rest: 70 seconds	
Week 2	Repeat 2 more times	Repeat 2 more times	
Week 3	20 reps each exercise	20 reps each exercise	
Week 3	Rest: 50 seconds	Rest: 50 seconds	
Week 3	Repeat 3 more times	Repeat 3 more times	
Week 4	15 reps each exercise	15 reps each exercise	
Week 4	Rest: 40 seconds	Rest: 40 seconds	
Week 4	Repeat 3 more times	Repeat 3 more times	
Week 5	10 reps each exercise	10 reps each exercise	
Week 5	Rest: 30 seconds	Rest: 30 seconds	
Week 5	Repeat 4 more times	Repeat 4 more times	

WORKOUT: LEVEL II

	Day 4 Thursday	Day 5 Friday	Day 6 Saturday	Day Sunday
	Cardio Warm-up	Cardio Warm-up	Cardio Warm-up	Off
	DB Chest Press ——— DB Lunge	Seated DB Shoulder Press ——— DB Pullover	DB Hammer Biceps Curl ——— DB Lying Triceps Curl	Off
	30 reps each exercise	30 reps each exercise	30 reps each exercise	
	Rest: 90 seconds	Rest: 90 seconds	Rest: 90 seconds	
	Repeat 2 more times	Repeat 2 more times	Repeat 2 more times	
	25 reps each exercise	25 reps each exercise	25 reps each exercise	
	Rest: 70 seconds	Rest: 70 seconds	Rest: 70 seconds	
	Repeat 2 more times	Repeat 2 more times	Repeat 2 more times	
	20 reps each exercise	20 reps each exercise	20 reps each exercise	
	Rest: 50 seconds	Rest: 50 seconds	Rest: 50 seconds	
	Repeat 3 more times	Repeat 3 more times	Repeat 3 more times	
	15 reps each exercise	15 reps each exercise	15 reps each exercise	
	Rest: 40 seconds	Rest: 40 seconds	Rest: 40 seconds	
	Repeat 3 more times	Repeat 3 more times	Repeat 3 more times	
	10 reps each exercise	10 reps each exercise	10 reps each exercise	
	Rest: 30 seconds	Rest: 30 seconds	Rest: 30 seconds	
	Repeat 4 more times	Repeat 4 more times	Repeat 4 more times	

(Continued next page)

5-FACTOR FITNESS

Day	Day 1	Day 2	Day 3
Phase/Time	Monday	Tuesday	Wednesday
Phase 4: Core 5 minutes	Upper-body Crunch	DB Lateral Flex/Extension	Off
Week 1	10 reps each exercise	10 reps each exercise	
Week 1	Rest: 10 seconds	Rest: 10 seconds	
Week 1	Repeat 4 more times	Repeat 4 more times	
Week 2	15 reps each exercise	15 reps each exercise	
Week 2	Rest: 15 seconds	Rest: 15 seconds	
Week 2	Repeat 3 more times	Repeat 3 more times	
Week 3	20 reps each exercise	20 reps each exercise	
Week 3	Rest: 20 seconds	Rest: 20 seconds	
Week 3	Repeat 3 more times	Repeat 3 more times	
Week 4	25 reps each exercise	25 reps each exercise	
Week 4	Rest: 25 seconds	Rest: 25 seconds	
Week 4	Repeat 2 more times	Repeat 2 more times	
Week 5	30 reps each exercise	30 reps each exercise	
Week 5	Rest: 30 seconds	Rest: 30 seconds	
Week 5	Repeat 2 more times	Repeat 2 more times	
Phase 5: Cardio 5 minutes (or more optional)	Cardio	Cardio	Cardio Optional

WORKOUT: LEVEL II (CONTINUED)

Day 4 Thursday	Day 5 Friday	Day 6 Saturday	Day Sunday
Lower-body Crunch	Upper-body Twists	Double-Crunch	Off
10 reps each exercise	10 reps each exercise	10 reps each exercise	
Rest: 10 seconds	Rest: 10 seconds	Rest: 10 seconds	
Repeat 4 more times	Repeat 4 more times	Repeat 4 more times	
15 reps each exercise	15 reps each exercise	15 reps each exercise	
Rest: 15 seconds	Rest: 15 seconds	Rest: 15 seconds	
Repeat 3 more times	Repeat 3 more times	Repeat 3 more times	
20 reps each exercise	20 reps each exercise	20 reps each exercise	
Rest: 20 seconds	Rest: 20 seconds	Rest: 20 seconds	
Repeat 3 more times	Repeat 3 more times	Repeat 3 more times	
25 reps each exercise	25 reps each exercise	25 reps each exercise	
Rest: 25 seconds	Rest: 25 seconds	Rest: 25 seconds	
Repeat 2 more times	Repeat 2 more times	Repeat 2 more times	
30 reps each exercise	30 reps each exercise	30 reps each exercise	
Rest: 30 seconds	Rest: 30 seconds	Rest: 30 seconds	
Repeat 2 more times	Repeat 2 more times	Repeat 2 more times	
Cardio	Cardio	Cardio	Off

· DAY 1: MONDAY ·

PHASE 1   Cardio Warm-up

PHASE 2   Strength Training: Dumbbell Chest Fly

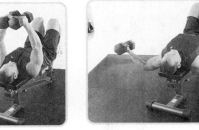

START   FINISH

PHASE 3   Strength Training: Dumbbell Tap Squat

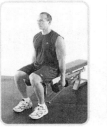
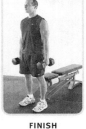

START   FINISH

PHASE 4   Core: Upper-body Crunch

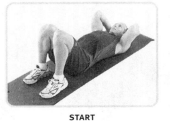
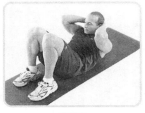

START   FINISH

PHASE 5   Cardio

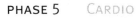

· DAY 2: TUESDAY ·

PHASE 1   CARDIO WARM-UP

PHASE 2   STRENGTH TRAINING: SINGLE-ARM DUMBBELL ROW

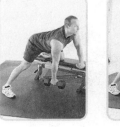

START   FINISH

PHASE 3   STRENGTH TRAINING: DB STIFF-LEGGED DEADLIFT

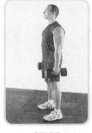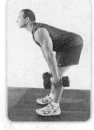

START   FINISH

PHASE 4   CORE: DB LATERAL FLEXION/EXTENSION

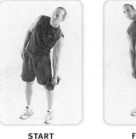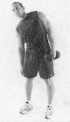

START   FINISH

PHASE 5   CARDIO

· DAY 4: THURSDAY ·

PHASE 1   CARDIO WARM-UP

PHASE 2   STRENGTH TRAINING: DUMBBELL CHEST PRESS

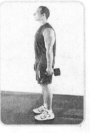 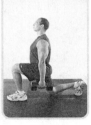

START   FINISH

PHASE 3   STRENGTH TRAINING: DUMBBELL LUNGE

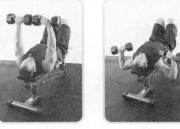

START   FINISH

PHASE 4   CORE: LOWER-BODY CRUNCH

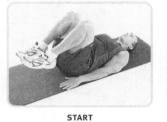 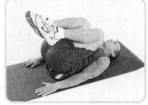

START   FINISH

PHASE 5   CARDIO

· DAY 5: FRIDAY ·

PHASE 1   CARDIO WARM-UP

PHASE 2   STRENGTH TRAINING: SEATED DB SHOULDER PRESS

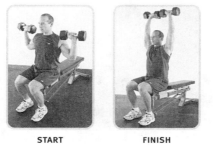

| START | FINISH |

PHASE 3   STRENGTH TRAINING: DUMBBELL PULLOVER

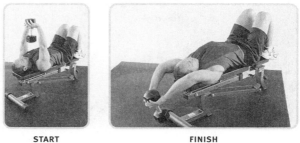

| START | FINISH |

PHASE 4   CORE: UPPER-BODY TWISTS

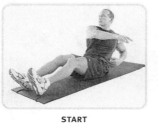 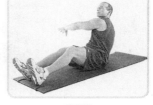

| START | FINISH |

PHASE 5   CARDIO

· DAY 6: SATURDAY ·

PHASE 1 CARDIO WARM-UP

PHASE 2 STRENGTH TRAINING: DB HAMMER BICEPS CURL

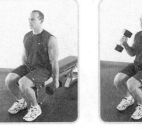

START   FINISH

PHASE 3 STRENGTH TRAINING: DB LYING TRICEPS EXTENSION

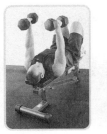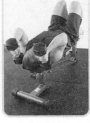

START   FINISH

PHASE 4 CORE: DOUBLE-CRUNCH

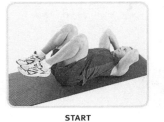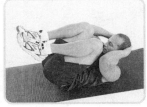

START   FINISH

PHASE 5 CARDIO

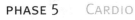

REAL RESULTS
Stephen Dorff • 36 • Actor

Just five weeks before a big studio movie production was set to begin, a producer called me up with a problem. The lead villain, to be played by Stephen Dorff, didn't resemble the physically intimidating character that had been written. Best known as the villain in *Blade,* Stephen was a skinny guy without much muscle tone. "Could you turn him into a chiseled, muscular antagonist in five weeks?" Armed with the 5-Factor program, I didn't hesitate: "Absolutely."

We didn't waste any time, as Stephen devoted himself to the program—never missing a workout and eating the 5-Factor way every day except Sunday (cheat day). Exactly five weeks later, he strutted onto the set ready for his series of shirtless scenes. The cast and crew were floored, for his body had transformed: suddenly he had muscles yet not an ounce of fat. Stephen himself had no idea his body was capable of looking that way, and he went on to use his fearsome physique to spectacular effect in the film.

After Week 5: What's Next?

When you've finished five weeks of level I, assess whether or not you are ready to move up to level II for the next five weeks. If you're already at level II, then simply repeat. Try increasing the resistance slightly on weeks six through ten.

Keep a good record of your workouts, so each month you can work toward increasing the poundages for each week's exercises as well as sticking to the suggested rep ranges and rest times.

PART

5-Factor Fuel

7 · Cutting Through the Fads and Hype

Whether you're conscious of it or not, the American food landscape is essentially a minefield—from ordering at a fast-food joint to the menu at a high-priced restaurant, from the vending machines and cafeterias at work and school to your very own kitchen. No wonder so many Americans are "blowing up" many sizes over what they should be. It's also no wonder why so many popular diet plans take an extreme approach to this landscape and essentially ask you to lop off a big portion of it, such as carbs, sugar, or calories.

Fortunately, the 5-Factor is not extreme in any way. I call it a "big picture" plan, which focuses on simple principles of good eating rather than counting carb grams or calories, or sending you shopping for exotic ingredients. Just as the fitness portion is more "doable" and "sustainable" than any other fitness plan out there, so is the food plan in relation to other books on the market. Everything is backed by solid reason and pure science.

5-Factor Nutrition

Scan any nutrition or diet section of a bookstore and you'll see how bewildering it is: eat for your blood type rather than your body type (*Eat Right 4 Your Type*); eat animal fats but almost no carbohydrates (*Atkins*); eats tons of salmon but no carrots (*The South Beach Diet*); eat grapefruits all day long (*The Grapefruit Diet*). From the cabbage soup diet to *The Zone,* I have read nearly every fad diet to be published over the past two decades. To some degree, all of these programs will help you lose weight in the short term. Yet, you often gain it all back, and then some, in the long term. What's more, in my opinion, none of them is good for your health or your enjoyment of life.

Many of today's popular diets are based on unsubstantiated theories, part-truths, and an "if something's good for you, then more must be even better!" attitude. As a result, we are yo-yoing our way from diet to diet in hopes of finding the secret way of eating that will enable us to look and feel eternally fabulous.

The premise of most recent fad diets (many of which are just the latest incarnations of fad diets from yesteryear) is weight loss through high-fat foods. Their argument is that carbohydrates do not fulfill your hunger and fat keeps you feeling full. The fuller you are, the less you will eat; and the less you eat, the more weight you will lose. While there is some truth to this, it is a gross oversimplification of a very complex process. It is simply not the whole story.

Many of these diets have capitalized on a particular problem: most people in modern society eat way too many simple carbohydrates (full of so-called "empty calories"), in the form of white bread, cake, cookies, French fries, chips, sugar-laden cereals, doughnuts, pizza, (overcooked) pasta, or all of the above in the same day; and even worse, some of these foods are high in fat as well. This leads, inevitably, to getting fatter, no question. Many of us know this, but why do we still stuff ourselves to the gills with this junk? One, it doesn't satisfy us for long, so we keep eating; two, we're conditioned to like it; three, it's everywhere.

Of course, too many such calorie-dense foods automatically add up to too many calories, subsequent weight gain, and often obesity. It's not an accident that, according to the Centers for Disease Control and Prevention, 64 percent of adults are obese or overweight; the number of overweight and obese youth has nearly doubled in the past two decades; and a poor diet—including obesity and physical inactivity—is about to overtake tobacco as the leading preventable cause of death in this country. Interestingly, these trends are mirrored in every other developed country, and even in some of the developing world. Meanwhile, obesity and inactivity contribute to the risks for some of the top killers: heart disease, cancer, stroke, and type II diabetes.

The trouble is, rather than educating the public on the differences between good and bad carbohydrates and teaching them the appropriate levels of good carbohydrates, many of these diet plans tell you to cut nearly *all carbohydrates* from your diet. Cutting out the major chunk of the average person's diet and going "low-carb" is essentially going "low-calorie," a far less attractive catchphrase. You better believe that these books wouldn't sell millions of copies if they admitted that fact and put "Low Calorie!" on the cover.

Cutting out a food group from your diet, of course, results in weight loss, so the low-carb locomotive continues to chug along. Besides making a demand that few people, no matter how disciplined, can stick to, here are some big problems with the low- or no-carb battle cry. Books like *Atkins* and *The Zone* aim to put you in a state called ketosis, which is actually a toxic state that ends up burning up fat but also your own body tissue, including muscle and even your organs. As soon as you introduce any significant carbohydrates, it stops working altogether. So on your one-week European vacation, by the fourth day, even though you're hitting the pavement for miles a day, you notice your face looking fuller and your pants feeling snug! Following a low-carb diet cripples your ability to exercise, if not sooner, then certainly later. Studies have shown that high-fat, low-carb diets deplete the stores of carbohydrates in your muscles and liver, which not only makes working out more grueling but even dangerous.* Additionally, your RPE (or rate of perceived exertion) is considerably higher on a low-carb diet than on a more moderate-carb eating plan. Eating a tremendous amount of fat and protein next to a scant amount of carbohydrates is not only unhealthy, it's also very difficult to put into practice. Last, just as your muscles require adequate carbohydrate intake to operate efficiently, so does your brain; so your mental skills will literally deteriorate if you follow a low-carb regimen.

*Jacobs, KA, DR Paul, RJ Geor, et al. "Dietary composition influences short-term endurance training–induced adaptations of substrate partitioning during exercise," *International Journal of Sport Nutrition and Exercise Metabolism* (2004) 14:38–61.

WHY FAD DIETS FAIL AND 5-FACTOR SUCCEEDS

1. They're unsustainable—5-Factor is easy to sustain week after week, year after year

2. They represent too big a departure from a normal eating style—5-Factor allows you to eat every type of food

3. They're often not healthy—5-factor is exceptionally healthy, emphasizing fibrous carbohydrates (including fruits and veggies), good fats, and lean protein

4. They're not accessible, requiring foods that are hard to come by—5-Factor's foods are easy to find and most of its recipes include only five ingredients

5. They require lots of prep time—most 5-Factor recipes take less than five minutes to prepare

6. They create a decrease in your daily performance, such as headaches, listlessness, and inability to concentrate—5-Factor will create more energy in you than you thought possible

REAL RESULTS
Jill • 37 • Real Estate Agent

A real estate agent in Toronto, Jill is a very busy woman and used to eat infrequently, often choosing nutritionally bankrupt foods. She exercised for one to two hours several days a week but was seeing no results: she had little muscle tone, a nagging shoulder injury, and lower back pain due to poor posture and significant muscle imbalances. While she was very logical and analytical with her business practice, this wasn't the case with her exercise and eating habits.

With 5-Factor, she radically redistributed her weight to the point that while she only lost 7 pounds, she went down *three dress sizes* in two months. Her posture significantly improved and she no longer had shoulder or back pain. She started eating five times a day, including between appointments with clients. Jill is proof positive that toning your body and redistributing weight can be just as dramatic as a large-scale weight loss.

8 · How 5-Factor Fuel Slims and Tones

Why five meals? Think of your body as a wood-burning stove: you have to stoke the fire early in the morning to warm up the house and continually feed the fire throughout the day to keep it warm. When nighttime arrives and everyone is set to go to sleep, you let the fire naturally burn down until morning, when you start the whole process over again.

Your metabolism works the same way. Start the day strong with a good 5-Factor breakfast, then periodically stoke your metabolic furnace during the day to keep it burning fat. Toward darkness, your body naturally slows down, and so should your intake until morning.

In the 1970s, researchers at the University of Toronto studied the effects of meal frequency on blood sugar and insulin secretion. They found that by eating many small frequent meals throughout the day, subjects were able to maintain stable blood sugar and insulin levels when compared to subjects who ate larger, less frequent meals. Referred to as "grazing" or "nibbling," the practice of eating many small meals a day was also shown to decrease levels of bad cholesterol.

Later studies actually found grazing to help in the reduction of body fat. Eating boosts the body's metabolism temporarily, which is called the thermal effect of food. The more meals a day, the more our metabolism surges.

With an increase in meal frequency also comes an increase in the control of the content and quantity of the food we eat. Today, unfortunately, most people starve themselves for periods of the day in which they often go five to twelve hours without eating anything. When they finally decide to eat, they have little control over what or how much they should eat—thus, their eating is driven mostly by hunger rather than foresight. Hunger is a very primitive drive that results from a physiological need to eat. When we eat frequent, smaller meals, we can decide what and how much to eat. This way, we are eating because we know it's a good idea to eat now, not because we desperately must eat something immediately.

Another reason that frequent, smaller meals are ideal is that we modern-day humans are physiologically identical to our caveman ancestors. As hunters and gatherers, they sometimes went for *days* without eating. Our species evolved the ability to shift into calorie-saving mode under such conditions, which allowed us to slow down our metabolisms and preserve our body's energy stores. This meant limiting the amount of our own body-fat stores that would be burned for energy, and also the additional food calories that came our way would be stored as body fat.

By eating frequently, we tell our bodies that we are living amid plenty and that we are in no danger of starving. This means that our body sidesteps the starvation/preservation cycle and our metabolisms are running "fast"; the wood-burning stove has enough wood coming in to keep the fire stoked and burning hot!

The 5-Factor's Five Keys to Fat Loss

The 5-Factor nutrition plan is based on science—hard, definitive, scientifically proven facts. Within this life-changing and body-bettering program, there are five keys for losing fat and/or gaining lean muscle, and you will assume control over every single one of them with 5-Factor:

1. *Metabolism:* As you probably know, the faster your metabolism, the more calories and fat you burn each day. How often you eat meals and whether or how often you do strength training determine how fast your metabolism is. The 5-Factor gets yours revving with five meals a day, every day, and ten minutes of strength training five days a week. For an analogy, look at a windmill: steady, regular gusts of wind make it turn at a good clip, but sporadic wind slows it down.

2. *Exercise:* Get into and stay in the fat-burning zone with cardio to nab that fat; meanwhile, strength-train to build lean muscle and up your resting metabolic rate so you literally burn more fat throughout the day, including while you sleep. A study published in the *Journal of the American College of Nutrition* showed that even people following an extremely low-calorie diet were able to increase their resting metabolic rate through the addition of strength training several times per week.*

*Bryner, RW, IH Ullrich, J Sauers, et al.; "Effects of resistance vs. aerobic training combined with an 800-calorie liquid diet on lean body mass and resting metabolic rate," 1999 Apr; 18(2):115–21.

3. *The right (kind and amount of) calories, naturally:* Rather than consuming foods that always leave you wanting more, you will eat good, healthy foods that fill you and provide the perfect level of calories per day for the weight you want to be (rather than drastically going under your caloric need, which many diets force you into and thus slow your metabolism down). The big bonus? You naturally will eat fewer calories per day than you presently consume, yet you won't have to count a single one.

4. *The glycemic index:* The GI will be explained below. It sounds daunting, but all it does is measure how much a carbohydrate food impacts your blood-sugar levels. High-GI foods raise your blood sugar, which then spurs the release of insulin and makes you vulnerable to storing these foods as fat; even worse, your hunger will continue to rage. However, low-GI, better foods keep your blood-sugar levels steady and you satisfied. Figuring out how to use the GI correctly can be the linchpin to losing weight.

5. *Rest and recovery:* To turn your body into an efficient fat-burning machine, your muscles need proper recovery for continual output and lean muscle gains. Proper rest and nutrition secure those needs. Meanwhile, two dominant hormones are affected by rest: growth hormone (especially in males) assists in lean muscle repair and building and is most active when you get proper rest. However, if you don't get proper rest, the "stress" hormone, cortisol, goes up and prompts greater fat storage.

It's no accident that four out of these five keys are heavily influenced by how you eat. If you read and follow the 5-Factor food plan, these four keys will be taken care of and you will be well on your way to a leaner, fitter body. The best news is that it isn't hard: just like you will always be able to find twenty-five minutes a day to do the 5-Factor workout, you will always be able to eat this way.

9 · Eating the 5-Factor Way

If the word "meal" frightens you because you're thinking, "How on earth can I prepare or consume five meals in one day?" think of it even more simply: you will eat the customary three meals (breakfast, lunch, and dinner) and two healthy snacks (in the mid-morning and the midafternoon). You'll see especially dramatic changes in your body if you have been one of those people who skips breakfast or doesn't snack between meals.

Asking you to eat the three standard meals of the day (breakfast, lunch, and dinner) with a snack in between them for a total of five times per day is not too great a departure from your normal routine, so you will be able to do it. If, on the other hand, I asked you to eat six or more meals a day, you may have to deviate significantly from your normal schedule. More important, you would have to deviate considerably from the schedule followed by your colleagues, whether they are your co-workers, fellow students, or family. We tend to take breaks at the same time as our colleagues. The norm is to take a break for lunch, plus a shorter break at midmorning and at midafternoon. Eating five meals a day fits perfectly into this schedule. We eat meal one before work and meal five after work. Meals two, three, and four are perfectly in sync with our predetermined work breaks.

How do the five meals relate to your sleep schedule? Simply, eat as soon as possible after you rise in the morning, whenever that is; and try to have the fifth meal a few hours before bed, whenever that is. (Aim for seven to eight hours of sleep for proper recovery and metabolic function.)

A nice perk of adopting this eating schedule is that you may well notice that your sleep improves. You will feel more energetic throughout the day and sleep more deeply at night. Also, if you have kids, they'll learn excellent eating habits and will get the same sleep benefits that you will. Remember how famished you were when you came home from school? If schools allowed kids fifteen minutes at midmorning for a snack, then they'd make better food choices at lunch and arrive home feeling good and interested in eating something small and nourishing, rather than tipping over the fridge and devouring its contents, assuming they didn't stop at a fast-food joint for a burger and fries first.

The Five Criteria per Meal

So, what should you eat? There are five simple criteria to follow when deciding on a meal.

1. Low-fat, quality protein

2. Low-GI carbohydrate

3. Fiber

4. Healthy fat

5. Sugar-free beverage

At every meal that you prepare, buy, or order, try to remember the five criteria of 5-Factor food. Here you're being handed the crucial knowledge of what makes up a balanced, nutritional, and flavorful meal—it's your road map. Whether your next meal is breakfast, a snack, or dinner, meeting these five criteria becomes easier and easier with practice. You will not have to sacrifice taste, quality, or certainly many varieties of foods. Yet you will gain a meal that will help you on your way to a lean, energetic body.

You will note that carbohydrates, protein, and fats represent three of the five criteria. These are also known as the three primary food groups, or macronutrients. *Carbohydrates* are the body's main source of fuel; they include all starches, sugars, and fiber. *Fat* has many functions; these include hormone regulation, body heat regulation, and organ insulation and protection. *Protein* forms the building blocks of the body's cells; it is the very fabric from which our skin, muscles, and red blood cells are made.

The U.S. government guidelines for macronutrient consumption are: 55 to 60 percent carbohydrate, 10 to 15 percent protein, and less than 30 percent fat. Popular diets such as The Zone (40/30/30) and Atkins advocate low levels of carbohydrate and much higher levels of protein and fat. Other diets, such as Pritikin (80/10/10) and Ornish (85/10/5), support very high intakes of carbohydrate with relatively minuscule levels of protein and fat. All have seen their days in the sun.

I recommend 55/30/15, and the suggested recipes roughly follow that design (and include the five criteria, of course); it essentially mimics the RDA for carbohydrate consumption but flips the protein and fat recommendations. However, now that you know the percentage breakdown, forget about it. Like I said at the top of the chapter, I don't want this to be an eating plan where you're weighing foods and counting grams, unless that's something you enjoy doing. For most people, tabulating total calories and percentages is tedious at best. Instead, I urge that you learn to "eyeball" your meals to make sure the three macronutrients roughly conform to these guidelines.

1. QUALITY PROTEIN

The need to ingest protein with every meal is a key component of the 5-Factor approach, for four reasons. First, compared to carbohydrates and fats, protein is very difficult to store as fat. We usually assimilate it, making it part of our lean body tissue, or excrete it.

The second reason protein must be ingested with every meal is that it cannot be stored and used later, unlike fats and carbohydrates. As a result, you must keep ingesting protein throughout the day so as to keep your body from breaking down your muscle and organs to meet its protein needs.

The third reason to consume protein frequently throughout the day is its metabolism-boosting effects. A great deal of recent research has shown that eating protein can actually kick-start your body's metabolism. Over the long haul, this can have a significant impact on your body composition, especially if you have been eating a lot of food: as you reduce your caloric intake and increase your exercise, consuming protein will help preserve your body's lean tissue (muscles as well as organs).

The fourth and final benefit of regular protein consumption is its ability to satiate. Protein makes you feel full—as, unlike many simple carbohydrates, protein can curb your hunger. For instance, eating bread without cheese, meat, or nut butter is a lot less filling and satisfying.

When deciding what type of protein to eat, you must take into account the fact that not all proteins are created equal. There are two key factors that determine the quality of a protein. The first is *bioavailability*: this is a measure of how much of a certain protein is broken down, absorbed, and assimilated into our body tissue. The more bioavailable the protein is, the less it travels through our system, failing to be absorbed, only to be excreted. The highest quality protein is whey. (In case you didn't know, whey is the murky translucent liquid that sits on top of yogurt; so the next time you open the carton, don't throw that away: stir it into the rest of the yogurt.) After whey come (in order) whole egg, milk, egg white, animal protein (chicken, fish, beef), soy, and vegetable protein.

The second factor determining the quality of the protein found in a given food is the degree to which it is *complete*. A complete protein contains all of the essential amino acids. Think of a protein as a train and the amino acids as the cars that make up the protein train. Protein is exactly that, a chain of amino acids. There are twenty-one amino acids. Most of the amino acids can be manufactured in the body. However, eight of them cannot. These eight must be ingested through food and are referred to as essential amino acids. If a protein has all eight essential amino acids, it is complete. For the most part, all animal sources of protein are complete. Vegetable sources of protein tend to be deficient in one or more amino acids.

For this reason, along with the greater bioavailability of animal proteins, it is simplest to go to animal-derived protein sources such as chicken, fish, beef, seafood, eggs, and dairy (milk, cheese, yogurt, and cottage cheese).

A caveat when consuming animal sources of protein is that you must watch their fat content. While some fat in the diet can be healthy, animal fat is not. Animal fat tends to be saturated and, therefore, may contribute to clogging of the arteries. So try to eat "clean" protein at every meal, and you will reap the benefits. No, it doesn't have to be ten egg whites or two chicken breasts like body-builders wolf down, but about a third to half of your meal should be made up of quality protein.

5-Factor Protein: Bacon and eggs, fried chicken, and sausage have a lot of protein, but they also have plenty of fat, most of it the artery-clogging, saturated kind. However, there are numerous all-protein foods that can be had in a variety of ways. Try to always have one of the foods listed below at each of your five meals.

1. Chicken (white breast meat, skinless)
   * Grill, BBQ, stir-fry, microwave

2. Fish (canned/fillets/steaks/raw)
   * Tuna or salmon salad (w/fat-free mayo)
   * Grill/bake fillets or tuna steak
   * Raw—sashimi, tartar, ceviche

3. Egg whites
   * Omelette, scramble, hard-boil

4. Cottage cheese (nonfat)
   * Plain or with fresh berries

5. Veggie meats
   - Hot dogs, deli slices, ground beef, bacon, burgers, pepperoni

6. Whey-protein shakes (low sugar)
   - With cold water (not milk); add ice and fresh fruit

7. Red meat (lean varieties of ground beef; top round, flank steak)
   - Grill, BBQ, stir-fry, microwave

8. Turkey (white breast meat, skinless)
   - Grill, BBQ, stir-fry, microwave

9. Seafood
   - Lobster, scallops, shrimp

10. Game
    - Bison, venison, ostrich

2. LOW-GI CARBOHYDRATE

When we consume too much carbohydrate, it suffers one of four fates: it is either used as an immediate energy source (such as a runner using Gatorade to increase glucose levels in the blood), stored as carbohydrate (in a form called glycogen), excreted (especially when it has a high fiber content), or converted to and stored as fat.

The glycemic index (GI) is a measure of your body's blood-sugar response to eating carbohydrate foods and was originally developed for use by type II (formerly known as "adult-onset") diabetics. Foods such as white bread and table sugar (sucrose) are at the top of the index, meaning that they have a value of 100. Eating these foods causes a sharp increase in blood sugar. With a sharp increase in blood sugar comes a corresponding increase in the hormone insulin; the presence of insulin makes us prone to store food as body fat. A chronic high level of insulin, hyperinsulinemia, is associated with type II diabetes, most of America's obesity, and even heart disease.* So our goal is to keep our insulin levels moderate by ingesting moderate- to low-GI foods.

Typically, foods that break down soon after you eat them get a high-GI number, while those that take longer to digest get a low-GI number. That's why a low-GI snack like cottage cheese and an apple will keep you from snacking again before dinner three hours later, while a couple of slices of white toast, or even worse, a bagel (which is also a calorie bomb), will soothe your hunger for only half that time or less. Going with low-GI meals helps your belly feel full earlier and stay full much longer, resulting in less overeating and better food choices. Because it doesn't cause blood-sugar spikes, you also get a steady supply of energy. With two brothers who are type I diabetics, I can tell you that if they don't have their regular small meals they get easily agitated, become irrational, and can't focus on anything! This is also what happens to low-carb dieters. Many of us are almost as strongly affected by the low blood-sugar phenomenon and may exhibit similar behavior when we've gone too long without food.

Just as protein and fat bring the GI number down, sugar increases it, which means that you must reduce your sugar intake if you want to lose fat. Not only does sugar contain many unnecessary calories, it raises your insulin levels and satisfies you only for a very brief period. You can't fool your body into treating 100 calories worth of lollipops the same way it handles 100 calories worth of an apple, just as you have always suspected.

*Willett, W, J Manson, S Liu. "Glycemic index, glycemic load, and risk of type 2 diabetes." *Am J Clin Nutr* 2002; 76:274S–80S.

While the glycemic index may appear complicated, principles that govern it are very simple. In particular, the following factors help keep the GI down and your blood sugar stable:

- *Fiber:* It prevents carbohydrates from being digested too rapidly (see fiber section on page 96).

- *Ripeness:* Ripe fruits and veggies have more sugar content than unripe ones (one of my favorite dishes at Thai restaurants is a green, or unripe, mango salad with chicken breast).

- *Type of starch:* Whenever you can, replace highly processed grains and cereals with minimally processed whole-grain products. Protein-enriched grains take half as long to convert to sugar in your blood compared to regular grains. (Lentils, wild rice, and quinoa are some of my favorite grains.)

- *Fat and acid:* The more fat or acid that a food contains, the more slowly carbs convert to sugar and are absorbed into the bloodstream. (It's why grapefruit and cherries are two of the lowest GI fruits.)

- *Firm, not soggy:* Cook vegetables and a starch like sweet potatoes to the point that it is just cooked—i.e., still a bit tough and chewy.

Here's a sampling of high-, moderate-, and low-GI foods (for more information, go to the GI database operated by the University of Sydney, Australia, at www.glycemicindex.com). Again, the lower the GI, the better the food is for you in terms of weight management.

Good GI Foods (Low to Moderate GI)	Bad GI Foods (High GI)
Steel-cut oats	Cream of wheat
Protein-enriched cereal	Puffed rice cereal
No-flour bread	White bread
Apple	Watermelon
Cherries	Dried fruits
Vegetables (almost all)	White potato
Nonfat plain yogurt	Tofu frozen dessert

The Forgotten Carbs: Fruits and Vegetables: With so many people eating on the run, ubiquitous high-protein or high-fat diets, and a preponderance of packaged foods, the mighty fruits and the valuable vegetable kingdom have been all but abandoned. This is a trend that I'd like to see you reverse—at least for yourself, if not for others.

Why? Well, for the normal reasons of good health—fruits and vegetables are chock full of essential minerals, vitamins, fiber, good carbohydrates, and phytochemicals. They also help lower your risk for certain cancers, stroke, heart disease, and high blood pressure.

Also, fruits and vegetables will help you lose weight for several reasons. One, they're accessible: easy to find and buy, and often easy to eat immediately. Two, they're fibrous. Three, they're low-glycemic. Four, they're water-based, so they take up a lot of room in your stomach and thus are filling, yet they are not calorie-dense. Five, making fruits and vegetables a part of your meals and snacks means that you're automatically cutting out less-nutritious foods: you don't see too many people having a papaya with a candy bar as a snack or some grapes and a piece of cherry pie after dinner. That candy bar and cherry pie suddenly aren't necessary when you get your taste buds to notice that there's nothing better than fresh, seasonal fruits and vegetables. Six, there are hundreds of varieties, so don't confine yourself to apples or oranges, or broccoli and lettuce. Constantly try new fruits and vegetables, and get into the habit of asking the produce person about what's fresh. Aim to get one to two servings of each per day.

3. FIBER

Fiber can actually help keep our blood-sugar levels stable. By slowing down the digestion rate of a meal, fiber ensures a gradual and steady release of energy into our system. Fiber has also been shown to help us feel full. Feeling full, or satiety, is an extremely necessary state of being when pursuing physique perfection. When we eat meals that do not satiate us, we tend to snack on unfavorable foods.

The health benefits of fiber are well established. Research has shown us that fiber can reduce the risk of developing various conditions, including heart disease, diabetes, bowel disorders, and certain cancers. Furthermore, fiber consumption can lower your blood-cholesterol levels.

Fiber is essentially carbohydrates that cannot be digested, and it's present in all plants that are eaten for food, including fruits, vegetables, grains, and legumes; and it is absent in animal foods, such as dairy, meat, fish, chicken, etc. Dietary fiber is the part of the plant-food source that your body cannot break down.

There are two kinds of dietary fiber: soluble and insoluble. Insoluble is popularly referred to as "roughage" and is not absorbed by the body, so it promotes good digestion and adds bulk to your stools; it's found in whole grains, vegetables, wheat bran, nuts, and beans. Soluble fiber draws water into your bowels, helping to protect you against bad cholesterol, heart disease, and colon cancer.

Sources include oats (especially oat bran), barley, beans, lentils, peas, nuts, seeds, apples and other types of fruits, and vegetables.

Fiber-Rich 5-Factor Foods: Currently, the recommendations for dietary fiber consumption are 20 to 35 grams per day; yet most Americans eat only half that amount. Here are some easy ways to get more fiber into your day:

- For breakfast cereal, choose only whole grain.

- Eat whole fruits (skins intact, when possible) instead of drinking fruit juice.

- Replace white or wheat breads with no-flour breads (much tastier than low-carb breads).

- Undercook rice, pasta, and potatoes so the texture is chewy rather than soft.

- Snack on raw vegetables (with skins intact, when possible— though you can still peel your carrots) instead of candy, chips, or crackers.

- From time to time, substitute low-fat legumes, like beans and lentils, for meat in chili and soups; or reduce the meat quantity in the recipe by two-thirds and replace with legumes.

Overall, rely on getting fiber from food sources rather than supplementing with fiber powders and the like.

4. GO LOW IN BAD FAT AND MODERATE IN GOOD FAT

For decades, the belief that the more fat you ate, the more body fat you stockpiled was shared by many nutritionists. We became "fat obsessed," and one trip down the supermarket aisle shows that we still are, with the preponderance of "fat-free" and "low-fat" items. Yet we as a nation are fatter than ever because these products may be low in fat, but they often are extremely high in sugar (to make them taste better) and thus calories, usually more than the full-fat versions that they are replacing.

Diets like Atkins and South Beach successfully challenged this formula and told you to eat fat—mostly because it helps you feel full. Yet many followers of the low-carb, high-fat regimen have gone the way of the successful low-fat, higher-carb dieters: weight loss in the short term (due mostly to fewer calories), then dissatisfaction with the diet coupled with diminishing returns leading to millions of dropouts.

As a result, going in the opposite direction and eating more fat than normal to lose weight doesn't work, either. One, fats are twice as calorically dense as carbs or protein, so in general you want to limit your overall consumption. Two, fats are also downright dangerous, as excess fat consumption has been shown to increase degenerative diseases (heart and arthritis), cancer, vascular disease (kidney and liver failure as well as stroke), heart attack risk, and even acne.

In particular, recent research implicates certain fats in the development of certain diseases. Saturated fats and especially trans fats worsen your blood-cholesterol levels and may pave the way to heart disease.

Saturated fats include mostly animal fats (such as meat, whole-milk dairy, butter, and egg yolks) as well as certain plant food (like coconuts, nuts, and palm oil); they raise both "good" HDL and "bad" LDL cholesterol (high-density lipoproteins, or HDL, make it less likely that excess cholesterol in the blood is deposited in the coronary arteries, while low-density lipoproteins, or LDL, carry cholesterol from the liver to the rest of the body and may deposit it on the walls of these arteries). Trans fatty acids (like margarine and French fries) are worse because they not only *raise* bad cholesterol but also *lower* good cholesterol. Avoid trans fats under all circumstances.

Some fats, meanwhile, can be good because they can actually improve blood cholesterol. These are unsaturated fats, including polyunsaturated and monounsaturated, that exist in plant sources like vegetable oils, nuts, and seeds. In addition, fats containing omega-3 fatty acids, like salmon and flaxseeds, are important; they make up nerve tissue, for example. Most American diets are woefully deficient in these fats, or even totally devoid of them. If you make sure to eat salmon, for instance, once a week (wild salmon is much lower in dangerous heavy metals than farmed salmon), that will usually be sufficient.

In general, the 5-Factor urges that you eat saturated fats sparingly and eat unsaturated fats in moderation for flavor and satiation. When eating meats, cheeses, and dairy, for instance, it is a good idea to go with low-fat or nonfat choices.

The Fat War: One of Good vs. Evil: Saturated fats can lead to many health problems, so minimize the intake of them as much as possible. Meanwhile, use moderate amounts of unsaturated fats in your diet to help lower cholesterol and satisfy your appetite. Often, you can substitute the latter fats for the unhealthy varieties by using olive- or canola-oil spray for sautéing rather than butter (certainly you should never use margarine, unless it's the kind you find at natural food stores that is unsaturated and is often bolstered by omega-3 fatty acids—ask for it).

"Good" Fats (eat in moderation)

Monounsaturated: avocado, canola oil, all or the majority of the fats in certain nuts (almonds, cashews, pecans, and peanuts), olive oil and olives, peanut butter and peanut oil, sesame seeds

Polyunsaturated: corn oil, cottonseed oil, safflower oil, soybean oil, sunflower oil, walnuts, pumpkin or sunflower seeds, mayonnaise, salad dressings, omega-3 fatty acids (albacore tuna, sardines, salmon, flaxseeds, etc.)

Bad Fats

Saturated (eat sparingly): whole milk, butter, cheese, and ice cream; high-fat red meat; chocolate; coconuts; palm oil; poultry skin

Trans (avoid at all costs): most margarines; vegetable shortening; "hydrogenated" anything, even partially hydrogenated vegetable oil; almost all commercially prepared baked goods, margarines, snack foods, processed foods, and commercially prepared foods, whether at the supermarket or in chain restaurants (like French fries)

5. SUGAR-FREE BEVERAGE

You know you should drink water (the standard recommendation is eight 8-ounce glasses a day, and more as needed after exertion and in hot or dry weather), but did you also know that drinking water can help you lose fat? It may have no calories, but having water between meals helps keep your stomach full. We have built-in sensors in our stomachs, so we get fuller sooner with liquid, which is also why soup is more filling than solid foods. So add a slice of lemon with some ice to your water for a pleasant variety once in a while.

There is some evidence, also, that when some people's bodies are craving water, it is read by their brains as a signal for sweets. Talk about crossed wires, right? If you seek that sweet thing in your mouth, choose sugar-free drinks that use Splenda (the safest, best-tasting sweetener) as the sweetener agent. Go with Hansen's natural diet sodas, Snapple's diet drinks, sugar-free lemonades (Crystal Light), sugar-free flavored waters, or ice teas. Of course, mineral and sparkling waters are always good. And skim milk is one of the perfect snacks. If you are lactose intolerant, you can go with a lactose-free skim milk. Occasionally, you can opt for the commercial diet soda, like Diet Sprite or Diet 7UP, both of which have no caffeine or artificial coloring.

What not to drink? Any liquid with sugar and/or lots of calories; any kind of juice is calorie-loaded and to be avoided; all milks except for skim have too much fat, most of which is unhealthy fat; soy milk is often high in fat and full of sugar, so look out; rice milk is all carbohydrates and sugar-laden; soda drinks are loaded with sugar and calories; sports drinks deliver calories you don't need unless you're a serious athlete; the multiple-calorie bombs served at java houses in which coffee is almost a minor ingredient; equally high in calories are seemingly-healthy-but-not juice shakes at certain places, which use sweeteners like sherbet (basically sugar) in most of their concoctions. Plus, because all the fiber has been sucked out as well as most of the vitamins and minerals, you lose the two most important parts of fruits with juice and only gain a ton of calories.

Staying away from such drinks will account for significant fat loss for some people who are used to having several hundred calories a day in liquid form alone.

Below is a list of standard drinks that many people consume on a weekly basis. If you consume *only one of each* at some point during the week, you would total 2,630 calories by week's end; and by year's end, you'd be at a staggering 136,760 calories.

Since 3,600 calories equal 1 pound of body fat, that equates to 38 pounds of extra fat. Scary, eh? That's why I endorse the sugar-free beverage.

Gatorade, 16 ounces = 100 calories

Wine, 5 ounces = 100 calories

Orange juice, 8 ounces = 110 calories

Rice milk, 8 ounces = 120 calories

Beer, 12 ounces = 150 calories

Coca-Cola, 16 ounces = 200 calories

Gin and tonic (2 ounces of gin) = 210 calories

White Chocolate Mocha at Starbucks, 16 ounces = 450 calories

Caribbean Passion at Jamba Juice, 32 ounces = 590 calories

Chocolate ice cream shake at Burger King, 16 ounces = 600 calories

Your Cheat Day

Sundays can be your "cheat day," during which you can eat what you want. Still try to stick to the five meals, and you won't overeat as much then, either. If anything, I've found that having a cheat day reinforces your discipline for eating well throughout the week. It's nice to know that you are not living in a food prison. But once you've had your fun, and maybe had too much cake or a massive steak, you may even realize that these forbidden foods weren't as delicious and delirious-making as you had once thought they were. They may even repel you during the week.

Plus, eating poorly for only one day is much better than eating "semi-poorly" every day, which describes many people's diets. One day of bad foods mostly goes right through you, while it's the accumulation of heavy, fatty, carb-crazy meals, day after day, that puts the love on the handles and the pot in the belly, bags in the saddles, and you get the idea!

Nutrition Q&A

Question: Are there any breads that are low-glycemic and that I can eat on this program?

Harley: I'm happy to report that, yes, there are. A few years ago, the average supermarket or even specialty shop carried no such breads, but times are changing. Essentially, the breads that qualify under 5-Factor are those that do not have flour as an ingredient, as flour simply acts like sugar in your bloodstream and wreaks havoc if you're trying to lose weight.

Breads such as Mestemacher and Ezekiel are made from whole-kernel grains, such as rye, wheat, or pumpernickel, and are not broken down like the typical bread. Fortunately, they also taste pretty good, but I recommend that you don't have more than one slice per meal, as I want you to get away from an overdependence on bread, such as always having to have a sandwich for lunch and toast with your breakfast.

Otherwise, try out brown-rice cakes as a "transport mechanism" for your protein. Use them with slices of chicken or turkey breast, nonfat cheese, veggie meats, or egg whites. They're airy and crunchy, so they fill your stomach and give you a pleasant texture, yet they do this without the calories and extra carbs (the average rice cake carries only 40 calories and 7.5 grams of carbs with it). Make sure there's no sugar (1 gram or less), especially no high-fructose corn syrup, and that they use brown rice (which is lower glycemic).

Another excellent transport are nonflour tortillas, rather than high-GI flour or whole wheat. Wrap one around some egg whites and salsa, or have one with sliced chicken breast and shredded nonfat cheese.

Question: I noticed on some package labels the term "net carbs." What does that mean, and is it a good thing?

Harley: A by-product of the low-carb movement, net carbs supposedly represent the total number of carbohydrate grams in a food product minus the grams of those carbs that cause little to no elevation in your blood-sugar level. Products that contain fiber, sugar alcohol (mannitol, sorbitol, xylitol, lactitol, isomalt, maltitol, and hydrogenated starch hydrolysates [HSH]), polydextrose, and glycerin, for example, appear to minimally affect your blood sugar, so the "net" carbohydrate total is calculated to be less than the "gross."

With so much venom directed at carbs in general, many product makers are now fond of using the term "net carbs" often with a single digit, such as "Only 7 net carbs!" Critics, however, say carbs are carbs, and any carbs that are consumed when your blood sugar is elevated will be stored as fat regardless of their propensity to raise or not to raise blood-sugar levels. Also, products that contain sugar alcohol commonly produce such unpleasantries as bloating and a laxative effect. (At press time, the FDA was investigating the entire low-carb labeling trend, including the "net carbs" claim.)

That being said, you will note that part of the purpose behind employing the glycemic index, as well as fiber, in the 5-Factor plan is blood-sugar control. As a result, I guess I could slap the "low net carbs!" label on the recommended 5-Factor foods or recipes—and fortunately that's without such awful-tasting and unnatural ingredients as stuff like sugar alcohol and glycerin.

Question: Should I eat any special way before or after a workout?

Harley: No, don't make it too complicated for you. Stick to the five meals per day; just make sure that you wait to exercise until at least an hour after you've eaten.

For the most part, the energy you draw upon for a workout under one hour is from the food you've eaten six hours or more ago, not recently, so don't chow down on a 300-calorie energy bar just before for a 300-calorie-burn workout.

Question: Are there any ingredients that I should avoid?

Harley: Most bad ingredients—such as saturated and trans fats like butter and partially or fully hydrogenated oils, as well as sugar—should be kept to a minimum in your diet, and now you probably can understand why. However, there is one incredibly common ingredient that you may not know too much about and it seems somewhat innocent, but you really should avoid like the plague: *high-fructose corn syrup.*

It's everywhere—in soft drinks, fruit beverages, cookies, jams, breads, ice cream, cakes, some crackers, spaghetti sauces, frozen pizzas, salad dressings, and on and on. Made from cornstarch, high-fructose corn syrup didn't even exist forty years ago, but more than 62 pounds of it was consumed per person in 2001 alone. It became popular to use by food manufacturers for three big reasons: one, it tastes sweeter than refined sugar, so they don't have to use as much (i.e., it's absurdly cheap and thus it saves them money); two, high-fructose corn syrup is easier to blend into beverages and foods than refined sugar; and three, it's cheaper to manufacture than refined sugar (again, saving them money).

But while it's an economical no-brainer for manufacturers to use the stuff, *it's a nutritional no-brainer to avoid high-fructose corn syrup.* Metabolically, it doesn't register in your body the same way that glucose does, but actually in a much more sinister way: it acts more like fat in terms of the hormones that are involved in potential weight gain. Fructose has also been shown to elevate levels of triglycerides and thus increase your risk for heart disease. This stuff never existed until very recently, and now it pervades the food supply, disturbingly, so be on your guard.

Question: Are there any supplements I should consider taking?

Harley: I get this question a lot from my clients, usually in relation to their desire to lose fat more quickly. I tell them that any product that tells you that it will fulfill that wish is not good for you. Also, 90 percent of supplements don't work and the few that do, the health risk is often too high. That means I advise against any kind of stimulant-based product, whether it's so-called "energy booster" drinks or capsules.

It's a matter of weight loss versus performance. If you can't do it for the rest of your life, then don't do it. Creatine, guarana, ephedrine? Nobody wants to take these products every day, which should tell you plenty. Having spent three years in a lab looking at ephedrine, I know it works, but I also know it can kill you: imagine redlining your car in first gear from L.A. to New York; it simply revs your body too high.

There are some standard supplements that I do recommend for everyone, and you can take them every day. The multivitamin/mineral (stick to one containing no iron if you are a man or if you are a woman who is no longer menstruating) provides the essential vitamins and minerals that you may not get from your daily food intake. They're a cheap insurance policy.

Meal replacements are not a necessity but are very convenient for those of you stuck at work, traveling, or are vegetarian or keeping kosher. They offer a tasty, quick, and simple way to get the right mix of protein, carbs, vitamins, and minerals you need without the hassle. They typically come in powdered packets; mix only with water, not juice or milk, to save the extra calories. Met-Rx, Myoplex, and Eat-Smart all make excellent meal replacements. They are available in supplement/vitamin stores, some grocery stores, and on the Internet.

You can also go with the even more convenient RTD (ready-to-drink) product, which is essentially a premixed liquid meal replacement in a bottle or can. Aim for one with less than 5 grams of sugar and little-to-no fat. Otherwise, you can use a quality whey-protein powder to mix with water; again, get one with low sugar. Put in a blender with ice, cold water, and some berries for a tasty, healthy snack or "dessert."

Whatever you choose for whey protein, you often don't want to follow the serving size, as it tends to be too large. Instead, aim for 20 grams of protein for women and 30 grams for men. Also, look for fiber as an ingredient in these whey-protein products.

Question: Should I be careful about my caffeine consumption?

Harley: Ah, caffeine, the most rampant addiction in the world. What with the ubiquitous Starbucks matching McDonald's, franchise for franchise, and Red Bull becoming de rigueur among the fashionable nightclubbing set, our caffeine-addicted nation shows no sign of slowing down. There's no doubt that it can keep you going when you would otherwise be flagging, but for the vast majority of us, it's something we use because, plain and simple, we're just addicted to it. When we don't have it, we get headaches; we feel drowsy; we get grouchy.

So I just say at least moderate your intake—such as a small cup of coffee in the morning after breakfast and maybe a cup of tea in the afternoon; that way, your level of addiction doesn't spiral out of control.

Going beyond that, such as downing Diet Cokes like water and clutching your cappuccino-to-go cup like it's a baby's bottle, is not advisable for several reasons. One, ramping up from a slight addiction to a major addiction means that you "can't get by without your fix" and start to rely on caffeine rather than your natural energy reserves. Plus, on days when don't get it, you suffer withdrawal symptoms and mood altering. Two, everyone has different levels of tolerance for caffeine, but it certainly affects your body's ability to recover, even if that means you can sleep but you may not sleep as deeply as you would without that after-dinner espresso; also, if you have heart issues, caffeine should be kept to a minimum (again, these issues could be latent, so proceed with caution).

Three, be aware that certain caffeinated drinks can be a Trojan horse of calories, with such calorific ingredients like whole milk, cream, sugar, chocolate, caramel, etc.; don't forget, the frappuccinos and mochaccinos taste so darn good because they're just loaded with sugar, fat, and calories! Replace that giant grande with a shot of espresso and skip all those calories; the 35 milligrams of caffeine are probably what you're after anyway.

10 · Your Daily Meal Plan

Let's go through a normal day and I'll show you where you can make better, more nutritional choices, without sacrificing taste or variety.

Breakfast

Cereal: skip the sugar-laden stuff and go with a cereal that has at least 5 grams of protein and 5 grams of fiber per serving, such as Kashi Go Lean! Toss in some fresh fruit, such as a few strawberries or some blueberries.

Want something warm instead of cold cereal? Use egg whites as a base for a low-fat omelette or simply scramble them up. Try the Apple-Cinnamon Oatmeal Frittata. (The recipe appears in the next chapter.) For hot cereal, make some oatmeal and blend in a scoop of whey-protein powder.

None of the above appeals to you? Then have a bowl of nonfat cottage cheese with a handful of berries thrown in.

Milk: for your cereal (cold or hot) or coffee/tea, skip the whole or percent varieties and use skim.

Optional sweetener: use aspartame or saccharine-free Splenda.

Optional toast: forget the white or wheat (which has a lot of white flour in it) breads and go with a no-flour bread. Its good taste will surprise you, and you'll find it much more filling.

Drink: water! Start hydrating yourself early in the day with water; after all, your body has probably just gone at least eight hours or more without it. Don't go the high-calorie juice route. Instead, get your fruit serving by having a whole piece of fruit (with skin and/or seeds).

Choose a sugar-free yogurt with berries, or have an apple with some cottage cheese. Blend up a shake with a handful of berries and a scoop of whey protein.

Lunch

Soups/salads: I'm a big fan of soups and salads, as they tend to be low in bad carbohydrates and can be chock full of vegetables and lean protein choices. As a result, they fill up your stomach nicely without an excess of calories. For soups, go with those using beans and good cuts of meat. For salads, choose ones with grilled chicken, tuna (even canned), or shrimp; top with one tablespoon of your favorite olive- or sesame oil–based dressing.

If a soup or salad doesn't do it for you today, you can have a sandwich with a few rules: forget the typical bun or bread, which are high-glycemic. Rather, use one slice of no-flour bread or a rice cake (see the bread question) to make an open-face lean meat (turkey or chicken breast, tuna, veggie meat, etc.) and optional nonfat cheese sandwich. Try the 5-Factor Reuben (recipe follows in next chapter). Or use a nonflour tortilla for a sandwich wrap. Add a slice of tomato and lettuce for extra bulk in your tummy.

Toppings: use mustard (Dijon or yellow) instead of calorific mayo, or ketchup/BBQ sauce (no more than one teaspoon because of the sugar) for extra flavoring.

Drink: have a diet drink, ice tea (with Splenda), or water.

Afternoon Snack

By this point in the day, you're understandably hungry, especially if you've already worked out. Rather than eating a bag of chips or a candy bar, give your body a nice variety of healthy yet tasty foods: a little nonfat cheese and an apple; a couple of dill pickles wrapped in turkey pastrami; a slice of nonflour toast with nonfat cream cheese, smoked salmon and sliced tomato; a rice cake with a slice of veggie salami and fat-free cheese; beef or turkey jerky with a piece of fruit.

Avoid so-called "protein" or "energy" bars. Typically, they're full of cheap ingredients like glycerin, bad fats, and high-fructose corn syrup. They may be "'high protein" but they're inevitably "high sugar" as well.

Dinner

Meat: pick a lean cut of protein, whether it's chicken, steak (small portion with no visible fat), or fish, and cook it with just half a teaspoon of olive or canola oil, such as when grilling, broiling, or microwaving. Add spices for extra flavoring.

Fibrous, moderate-GI carbohydrate: steer away from fatty, high-glycemic typical carb sides like potatoes, pasta, or rice. Instead, go with wild rice, squash, sweet potato, or a vegetable, such as broccoli, spinach, or cauliflower. Try a one-pot meal such as the Cioppino or HP's Big City Chili. (Recipes follow in next chapters.)

Drink: most are tempted to have something calorific, from soda to beer suds, at this hour; instead, stick with water or have some Crystal Light or Hansen's Diet (all without caffeine) soda.

Meal Plans

Here are some sample meal plans to help you get started. The 5-Factor plan leaves plenty of room for flexibility. Most of the suggestions below are easy to prepare in five minutes or less.

5-Factor Sample Meal Plans

· MONDAY ·

MEAL	NAME	PROTEIN	CARBOHYDRATE
1	Apple-Cinnamon Oatmeal Frittata	(egg whites)	oatmeal, dried apples
2	Snack	nonfat cottage cheese	apple
3	Curried Chicken Salad*	chicken breast nonfat yogurt)	slice of no-flour bread
4	Snack	veggie salami nonfat cheese	Brown rice cake
5	Lemon Salmon*	salmon	quinoa, side salad

· TUESDAY ·

MEAL	NAME	PROTEIN	CARBOHYDRATE
1	Cereal	skim milk	Kashi Go Lean! Cereal
2	5-Factor Protein Shake*	whey protein	frozen berries
3	HP's Big-City Chili*	lean ground beef	mixed bean stewed tomatoes
4	Snack	smoked salmon nonfat cream cheese	slice of no-flour toast
5	Dinner	grilled chicken breast	wild rice, broccoli

* These recipes appear on the following pages.

· WEDNESDAY ·

MEAL	NAME	PROTEIN	CARBOHYDRATE
1	5-Factor Frittata*	egg whites, nonfat cheese, chicken	bell pepper
2	Cinnamon Apple Treat*	nonfat yogurt	apple
3	5-Factor Reuben*	turkey pastrami nonfat cheese	sauerkraut no-flour bread
4	Snack	jerky (beef, turkey, or salmon)	piece of fruit
5	Asian Wraps*	ground chicken breast	shiitake mushrooms Boston lettuce

· THURSDAY ·

MEAL	NAME	PROTEIN	CARBOHYDRATE
1	5-Factor French Toast*	egg whites, nonfat milk	2 slices no-flour bread
2	Snack	nonfat yogurt	peach
3	Turkey Stew*	turkey breast	sweet potatoes tomatoes
4	Thai Egg Strips*	egg whites	shallot, scallion, red chili
5	Dinner	fillet of tilapia	spaghetti squash side salad

· FRIDAY ·

MEAL	NAME	PROTEIN	CARBOHYDRATE
1	Cereal	skim milk	Kashi Go Lean! Cereal
2	5-Factor Berry Shake*	whey protein	frozen berries
3	Chef Salad*	turkey breast, boiled egg whites, nonfat cheese	romaine lettuce
4	Snack	nonfat French onion/ sour cream dip	celery sticks
5	"I can't Believe It's Not Pizza" Pizza*	veggie pepperoni nonfat cheese	flourless wrap tomatoes

· SATURDAY ·

MEAL	NAME	PROTEIN	CARBOHYDRATE
1	Breakfast Burrito*	egg whites, veggie bacon, nonfat cheese	flourless wrap, salsa
2	Snack	nonfat cottage cheese	pear
3	Mediterranean Tuna Salad*	albacore tuna, chickpeas	tomato, lettuce
4	Snack	turkey breast slices nonfat cream cheese	lettuce, green pepper
5	Dinner	grilled chicken breast	sweet potato, peas

· SUNDAY ·

Free day! Eat whatever and whenever you want, and eat as much as you want.

5-Factor Eating Tips

Be proactive, not reactive, with your diet. You make bad choices with food and drink when you don't have a game plan and are tempted by anything that's waved in front of your face. Follow the tips below, and making good choices will become automatic.

CLEAN HOUSE

Here's the number-one tip, and it may be a hard one to swallow. I recommend that you get rid of all the junk in the shelves, fridge, and freezer. What am I talking about? The sugary cereals, white bread, chips, cookies, etc. Replace them with healthier varieties the next time you go shopping. In general, try to buy more "real food"—meats, dairy products, whole grains, fruits, and vegetables—rather than mostly packaged goods. Remember, anything that says "hydrogenated" or "high-fructose corn syrup" on the label is to be avoided. The pounds will come off faster and faster, just as soon as you put better food in the house.

GETTING BY ON LESS

If you're used to eating a lot of bad calories, the first few days may be difficult to get through without sneak-snacking outside the five meals. That's your body trying to get your fat back! Fight through the urge, or nibble on something very healthy. Distract yourself with something completely unrelated to food, and the urge to gorge will likely pass. The interesting phenomenon noted by my clients, myself, and others is that when you work out five days a week, your appetite actually is moderated rather than increased! That seems totally counterintuitive, but it's true. Part of it is psychological: because of the workouts, your body starts to look better and you start to feel better as well; you then develop a natural urge to take care of your body rather than go down the road of sabotage.

GO ONCE, GO SLOW

Fill your plate once, and fill it thoughtfully with different colors, textures, varieties. Then don't fill it again. When you start to eat, go slowly and enjoy. This seems simple, but it bears repeating because it can be hard to put into practice consistently. Remember, as you get older, you eat less but enjoy it more. If possible, try eating with a friend, colleague, or other good soul who enjoys conversation. The more you talk and are enjoying the other person, the less quickly and less quantity you'll eat.

DOWNSIZE

If you want to shrink your fat cells, then you also have to shrink the objects that you eat and drink from. From plates to bowls to soda containers to wine glasses, everything is bigger—and thus so are the portions. Because we're conditioned to "clean our plate," we do so, even if it's enough food to feed two. People in generations past were smaller in part because they never used such monster-size dishes, glasses, and containers. So it's no wonder our generation is the fattest in human history.

Fight the tide by purchasing more reasonable-sized dishes, glasses, and containers, which will help reinforce that you consume more reasonable-size portions. And always use these dishes, rather than eating out of large containers, such as a bag of chips or pint of ice cream.

Away from home, be wary of the huge portions they love to serve you at restaurants, from high-end to fast food, and either order less or take part of it home in a doggie bag. Only recently, McDonald's made the unexpected and impressive move to remove the "supersize" option from their menu; while their food mostly remains suspect, even at places like McDonald's you now can have a meal that resembles 5-Factor and fulfills the five criteria (such as a grilled chicken breast, a side salad, low-fat dressing, and Diet Coke or a bottle of water).

CLEAN YOUR PLATE IN THE SINK, NOT YOUR MOUTH

Ever notice that some people always leave a few bites on their plates (generally slim people), and that others never do, even when they complain how their full stomachs are starting to ache? It comes down to the messages they got in their earliest childhoods from their parents and caretakers. In some households, leaving something on your plate was a grave offense; in others, it elicited no comment whatsoever. Some kids are praised for finishing their food and cajoled endlessly to eat more; others are left alone in this regard. Whatever happened to you at a young age, you are a mature person now who has the power to or not do things, according to your own will. Claim that power, and use it.

ISOLATE TO OVERCOME

Isolate the parts of the day when you make poor food choices; rather than just saying, "I will be strong and not do that again," learn from the experience and *plan* to eat a better food next time. The periods of late afternoon to the pre-dinner period and the late night are the two toughest times of day, when the "munchies" can grab you. Anticipate it by having a 5-Factor snack, such as a whey-protein shake with berries or a piece of no-flour toast with some nonfat cream cheese. Your body naturally wants food every three to five hours that you're awake; respect its wishes or you will cave in to the cravings.

HANDLE THE HUNGER

Eating five meals a day will usually work to keep hunger at bay, but occasionally it will rage without too much warning. Hunger is a signal that your body gives your brain because it is searching for nutrients; so go the healthy route and give it what it's really looking for. Empty calories don't do much to calm your hunger. After your hunger is appeased with healthy foods eaten at regular, reasonable intervals, then you can eat the occasional not-so-healthy stuff with much more discipline and moderation, instead of bingeing.

FILL THE VOID, NOT YOUR FAT STORES

Stress, boredom, and unhappiness are three big reasons for eating poorly, but such "states" require much better solutions than calories. Rather, being active (including doing the 5-Factor workout) will do much more to alleviate those problems.

HAVE A PLANNED "SIT-DOWN"

Did you know that your body doesn't register that you're consuming calories as much when you're standing versus sitting down? (Now you know why you can eat hors d'oeuvres at a party all day long without noticing.) So try to cut out the stand-up snack or must-sample-while-cooking routine and wait to eat until you sit down.

Additionally, develop a routine in which you sit down for those five meals at approximately the same time every day, as your body will naturally adjust to this pattern and will learn to be less hungry during the in-between times. A sample day of eating times could be: 7 A.M., 10 A.M., 1 P.M., 4 P.M., and 7 P.M.

PREVENTING "PARENT FAT"

For many people, becoming a bigger family becomes a reality, literally. Whether it's one kid or several, parents don't have as much time to exercise, and their meals suddenly revolve around their children's. Both can mean double trouble for our waistline. Common habits develop, such as finishing whatever your child does not (those calories actually do add up!), catering to your child's demands to prepare junk foods like hot dogs and macaroni and cheese, and eating at tons of fast-food joints and "family restaurants" that treat grease like an essential fatty acid and beg you to load up, because after all, it's "all you can eat."

Besides losing these bad habits, make your 5-Factor food and workouts a priority, thus developing a higher level of energy and setting good examples for your children.

DESSERT

If you can go without these extra sweet calories at the end of the day, do so. Or if a nice mixture of fruit does it for you, do that. Remember, you have the "cheat day" on Sunday to enjoy a richer dessert.

For some of us, however, we have days when dessert after dinner is something we don't want to go without. Try sugar-free, fat-free varieties of ice cream, frozen yogurt, pudding, and Jell-O, although I caution you against forming an excessive dependence on artificial sweeteners. It's far easier to quell sugar cravings when your taste buds have become less accustomed to the sensation of sweetness, and I don't recommend using artificial chemicals in large quantities in your food or drink.

STOP AND SMELL THE ROSES

This phrase is packed with wisdom, and the special meaning it conveys to us in this regard is "Remember to stop and breathe." It's easy for some people to go a whole day running around in a frenzy without taking even one good, deep, belly-filling and belly-emptying breath. Obviously, 5-Factor Fitness will get you breathing, but you need to do it the rest of the day, too, when you are able to grab whatever food you crave (you don't live in the Amazon basin, so it's a reality, even though you won't be stocking inferior foods at home).

If you're the type of person who eats "to relax," then you may well benefit hugely from remembering to do this—while eating, one does breathe deeply, and thus, one feels calmer (the same is true of smoking, which is another insidious habit, one that is even more deleterious to your health). In times of stress, we breathe shallowly (an adaptive response that helped our distant ancestors, who had to be ready to take flight or to fight); at the office, you aren't going to run away or get into a battle (although you may sometimes be tempted to do both!), so you don't benefit from breathing shallowly. In fact, deep breathing will prevent a whole host of physiologically undesirable responses from being triggered, such as the secretion of cortisol in your blood. In any case, you won't fall prey to the urge to keep a bag of chocolate chip cookies or caramels in your desk drawer "for emergencies."

A LABEL LOOK-SEE

When you buy packaged goods, don't just glance at the commercial side of the package that tells you how great their product is. Flip it over and take a close look at the nutritional label. In particular, look for these things:

- *Serving size:* many manufacturers choose absurdly small serving sizes to make the calorie, fat, and carb counts seem little. First, estimate the fat and carbohydrate grams of a real serving of this food, using the proportion of each in their "serving size."

- *Calories:* next look at the calories in a "real serving." If it's a frozen entrée, then it shouldn't go above 350 calories; if it's a snack, 150 calories is about right.

- *Carbs/protein/fat:* rather than look at each one individually, look at them collectively. Aim for a "macronutrient" combination, so you get a balanced blend of the three; go a little higher in carbs and moderate in protein and fat. Avoid the all-carb packages; you must have protein and fat in there to create satiety.

* *Sugar/fiber/saturated fat:* under the carbohydrates listed, check to see how much sugar is in the product; if it goes over 10 grams, then that's too much (many "healthy" energy bars have more than 15 grams of sugar). Also listed under carbs is the fiber content; try to get some fiber in all packaged goods that you purchase. Under fat, note how much saturated fat it has; aim for little to none.

* *High-fructose corn syrup/hydrogenated oils:* if either of these two are on the list of ingredients, put it right back on the shelf.

REAL RESULTS
Kathyrn Garcia • 53 • Registered Nurse

When Kathryn started on the 5-Factor, she weighed almost 200 pounds, even though she went for a one-hour walk each morning. As a result of the excess weight, she had horrible knee problems that impacted her job performance. She was also very unhappy in her personal life and had recently been divorced.

Kathryn's first question for me was about the diet plan. She'd tried plenty of programs and always ended up caving in to her food cravings. She was thrilled at the prospect of being able to eat five meals a day and still lose weight. Kathryn embraced the 5-Factor method wholeheartedly, and she let it turn her life around. Her weight dropped to 138 pounds, while her confidence soared to the point that she started dating again.

11 · The 5-Factor Recipes

Maybe you can only cook scrambled eggs. Or you're as comfortable cooking Cantonese as you are cooking Cajun. Either way, the 5-Factor food recipes will surprise you: not only are they easy to put together as well as flavorful, but they will help you with your goals of losing fat and/or gaining lean muscle.

Each meal represents total nutrition, with the five criteria included: (1) a low-fat protein source, (2 and 3) a fibrous low-glycemic carbohydrate, (4) a good fat source, and (5) a no-sugar drink.

The number-one reason people claim they are unable to prepare their own meals, and therefore eat healthfully, is lack of time. We often don't have an hour to prepare a meal; we also sometimes struggle to make something that's healthy *and* satisfying in a short amount to time. Using a few shortcut tricks, I'll show you how you can cut meal preparation time way down so it's no longer an excuse not to eat well.

The truth is that most dishes can be made simply and deliciously using only five ingredients and taking only five minutes to prepare.

We designed these recipes to be as easy as possible, but if you don't want to use the microwave, you can prepare most of them on the stovetop. If you wish to use dried beans rather than canned, you can take the time to soak them overnight. The eating plan is meant to be flexible, and within that spirit I encourage you to develop your own 5-Factor recipes and feel free to share them with me at www.5factorfitness.com.

Remember, it is crucial to eat five modestly sized meals per day in order to stoke your metabolism, maintain a good energy level, and help your body recover from the workouts—all of which lead to a leaner, firmer physique.

Meal 1: Breakfast

The most important meal of the day, your breakfast should be eaten soon after you get out of bed (like before you jump in the shower—save that for after you've fueled up) to get your fat-burning metabolism going. There are always high-protein/low-sugar cereals such as Kashi Go Lean!, oatmeal with skim milk, or egg whites and a slice of no-flour toast.

Otherwise, try these recipes:

Breakfast Burrito

SERVES 1

4 egg whites (from carton)
4 *Yves* Veggie Bacon Strips, diced
1 large flourless wrap (Ezekiel)
½ cup nonfat cheese
1 to 2 tablespoons salsa

Spray a medium-size omelette or frying pan with canola oil spray.

Cook the eggs and veggie bacon in the pan over medium heat for 2 minutes, stirring to scramble.

Place the eggs and veggie bacon in the wrap and immediately cover with shredded nonfat cheese. Add 1 or 2 tablespoons of salsa, and roll up to serve.

Apple-Cinnamon Oatmeal Frittata

SERVES 1

4 egg whites (from carton)

½ cup rolled oats

2 to 3 tablespoons diced dried apples

1 teaspoon cinnamon

2 tablespoons unsweetened, natural applesauce
   (for garnish)

Spray a shallow microwave-safe bowl with canola oil for 1 second.

Pour egg whites into the bowl. Stir in oats, dried apples, and cinnamon.

Cover with plastic wrap, venting one side, and microwave on High for 3 to 4 minutes until egg whites are firm. (Alternatively, this can be cooked on the stovetop in a skillet like a pancake.) Top with applesauce and serve.

Open-Faced Breakfast Sandwich

SERVES 1

4 egg whites (from carton)

4 *Yves* Veggie Back Bacon

2 slices of nonfat cheese (cheddar, Swiss, etc.)

1 slice no-flour bread, cut in half, or rice cakes

1 slice tomato

Spray a shallow microwaveable bowl with canola oil spray for one second. Pour the egg whites into the bowl and microwave on High for 3 to 4 minutes until firm.

Grill the Veggie Back Bacon in a skillet for 2 minutes or place in a microwave-safe dish and microwave on High for 1 minute.

Cut the cooked egg whites into four wedges. Place two wedges of egg white, one slice each of bacon, and cheese on each half slice of bread or rice cake and serve.

Power Porridge

SERVES 2

½ cup rolled oats

3 cups water

1 cup chopped fresh/frozen fruit (berries, peaches, apples)

1 teaspoon apple-pie spice

1 teaspoon vanilla

1 tablespoon Splenda

Put the oats, water, fruit, spice, vanilla, and Splenda in a microwave-safe bowl. Cover, venting one side, and microwave on High for 2 minutes. Stir and microwave for 1 to 2 minutes, until thickened and bubbly.

5-Factor Frittata

SERVES 1

½ cup chopped onion
½ cup chopped bell pepper (any color)
4 egg whites (from carton)
½ cup shredded nonfat cheese (mozzarella, Swiss,
   cheddar)
2 slices smoked chicken or turkey breast, chopped

Spray a wide, shallow microwave-safe bowl with canola
oil spray. Add the onion, bell pepper, and egg whites to the
bowl. Cover with plastic wrap, vented on one side. Microwave on High 3 to 4 minutes until egg whites are firm.
Remove from microwave and immediately top with cheese
and meat.

Serve with a slice of no-flour toast.

Italian Omelet

SERVES 1

4 egg whites (from carton)
1 Roma tomato, chopped
½ small zucchini, finely chopped
1 teaspoon dried basil
½ cup chopped bell pepper (any color)
½ cup shredded nonfat mozzarella cheese

Spray a wide, shallow microwave-safe bowl with canola oil spray. Add the egg whites, tomato, zucchini, and basil to the bowl and mix to combine. Cover with plastic wrap, venting one side. Microwave on High for 3 to 4 minutes until the egg whites are firm. Remove from microwave and immediately sprinkle with the cheese. (Serve with a slice of no-flour toast.)

French Toast

SERVES 1

4 egg whites (from carton)
½ cup nonfat milk
½ teaspoon ground cinnamon
1 teaspoon vanilla extract
2 slices no-flour bread

Mix the egg whites, milk, cinnamon, and vanilla in a medium-size bowl. Spray a wide, shallow microwave-safe bowl with canola oil spray. Place the bread in the bowl in a single layer. Pour the milk mixture over the bread and turn to coat the bread on all sides. Cover with plastic wrap, venting one side, and microwave on High for 2 to 3 minutes until cooked through. (Garnish with berries and serve with sugar-free pancake syrup if desired.)

5-Factor Scramble

SERVES 1

½ cup chopped onion

4 egg whites (from carton)

½ cup cooked ground chicken or turkey breast

½ Roma tomato, chopped

½ cup sliced mushrooms

Spray a wide, shallow microwave-safe bowl with canola oil spray. Add all the ingredients to the bowl. Cover with plastic wrap, venting on one side, and microwave on High for 3 to 4 minutes until the egg whites are firm. Season with chopped fresh cilantro, if desired, and serve with a slice of no-flour toast or a no-flour tortilla.

Meal 2: Midmorning Snack

Between your breakfast and lunch, get in a worthwhile snack to keep your blood-sugar level stable and metabolism humming. Pieces of fruit with nonfat cottage cheese, nonfat plain yogurt with fresh fruit, or an easy-to-make 5-Factor berry shake are good morning snacks. Here are some special recipes worth trying:

Apple and Ricotta

SERVES 1

1 apple, chopped
½ cup nonfat ricotta or cottage cheese
½ teaspoon cinnamon
1 packet Splenda
1–2 tablespoons unsweetened apple sauce

Mix the apple, ricotta or cottage cheese, cinnamon, and Splenda until thoroughly blended. Serve topped with apple sauce.

Cinnamon Apple Treat

SERVES 1

1 apple (Granny Smith works best)
½ cup nonfat plain yogurt
1 teaspoon cinnamon
1 packet Splenda

Core the apple and place in a small, microwave-safe bowl. Add remaining ingredients. Microwave on High for 4 minutes.

5-Factor Berry Shake

SERVES 1

8 ounces cold water

1 to 2 scoops (approximately 7 tablespoons) whey or soy
protein powder (MetRx, Myoplex, Eat Smart, or any
protein powder with less than 5 grams sugar per
serving)

1 cup frozen berries (strawberries, blueberries, black-
berries, raspberries)

1 cup ice cubes

Put all the ingredients into a blender. Process on High
until berries are pureed.

Meal 3: Lunch

The most common lunch is a sandwich. In 5-Factor, you should go
with a lean meat, such as turkey breast, then add some nonfat
cheese, and add a slice of tomato for nutrients. Since you're having
bread, you're already getting plenty of carbohydrates, so you can
lose the extra carbs of chips or fries, which are often served with a
sandwich. Have a salad—use only 1 tablespoon of your favorite
olive- or sesame oil–based dressing, rather than fat-loaded cream

dressings or sugar-loaded nonfat dressings. Add a piece of fruit, such as an apple, and have that first, to lower the GI of the meal.

When you need a change from the boring old sandwich routine (and you will), here are some great lunches you can make up quickly:

Curried Chicken Salad

SERVES 1

½ pound cooked chicken breast, chopped
¼ onion, diced
½ cup plain nonfat yogurt
1 tablespoon curry powder
2 ounces water

Mix all the ingredients in a microwave-safe bowl. Cover with plastic wrap, venting on one side. Microwave on High for 1 to 1½ minutes. (Serve open-faced on a single slice of no-flour bread or on a bed or romaine lettuce.)

Tuna Lettuce Wraps

SERVES 1

1 6-ounce can water-packed tuna

¼ cup chopped tomato

¼ cup chopped celery

1 tablespoon nonfat mayonnaise

2 to 4 leaves of iceberg lettuce

Mix the tuna, tomato, celery, and mayonnaise in a bowl until combined. Season with pepper. Spoon the tuna mixture into the lettuce leaves and wrap to enclose filling.

HP's Big-City Chili

SERVES 4

2 pounds ground chicken or turkey breast

1 15-ounce can stewed tomatoes (Mexican-style if
  possible)

1 15-ounce can mixed beans (e.g., kidney, garbanzo,
  black, etc.)

1 6-ounce can tomato sauce (no sugar added)

1 tablespoon chili seasoning

Brown the chicken in a medium-sized pot over medium
heat, stirring to break up the meat. Add the remaining ingredients and stir. Bring to a boil, reduce heat, and simmer
for 5 to 15 minutes to combine flavors.

5-Factor Reuben

SERVES 1

1 to 2 teaspoons nonfat Russian dressing

2 to 4 tablespoons sauerkraut, drained

1 slice no-flour bread

4 to 6 slices turkey pastrami

1 to 2 slices nonfat cheese

Spread Russian dressing and sauerkraut on bread. Put the turkey pastrami on top of the sauerkraut and then add the cheese on top of the pastrami. Place under a broiler for 4 minutes or microwave on High for 50 seconds to 1 minute. Season with pepper. Serve with a dill pickle.

Cajun Red Beans and Rice

SERVES 2

½ cup chopped red onion

1 15-ounce can red beans

1 15-ounce can diced tomatoes

1 package *Yves* Veggie Dogs, chopped

1 tablespoon Cajun spice blend

Spray a wide, shallow microwave-safe bowl with canola oil. Add all the ingredients to the bowl. Cover with plastic wrap, venting on one side. Microwave on High for 4 to 5 minutes, until bubbly.

Serve each portion over ½ cup cooked brown rice or quinoa. Garnish with dried parsley and cilantro.

Turkey Stew

SERVES 2

1 pound turkey breast tenderloins, chopped

1 large sweet potato, diced

1 medium red onion, sliced thin

1 14.5-ounce can crushed tomatoes with Italian
    seasoning

2 teaspoons minced garlic

Spray a wide, shallow microwave-safe bowl with canola oil. Add all the ingredients to the bowl. Cover with plastic wrap, venting on one side. Microwave on High for 4 to 5 minutes. Stir, re-cover, and microwave on High until turkey is cooked through and sweet potato is tender.

"I Can't Believe It's Not Pizza" Pizza

SERVES 1

1 large flourless wrap (Ezekiel)
3 tablespoons (Arrabiata, marinara, or other)
    tomato sauce
1 Roma tomato, sliced
6 slices *Yves* Veggie Pepperoni
½ cup shredded nonfat mozzarella cheese

Place the wrap flat on a ridged skillet (a flat skillet will also do, as will a grill). Spread tomato sauce on the wrap.

Add the sliced tomatoes, pepperoni, and mozzarella on top of the marinara sauce. Cook over low to medium heat until cheese melts, about 2 minutes. Slice into wedges.

Chef Salad

SERVES 1

¼ pound smoked turkey breast

2 hard-cooked egg whites

3 to 5 leaves romaine lettuce, torn into bite-size pieces

½ cup shredded nonfat cheese (cheddar, mozzarella, or
   Swiss)

1 to 2 tablespoons nonfat Thousand Island dressing

Chop the turkey breast and egg whites. Place the lettuce in a bowl. Top with the turkey, egg whites, and cheese. Add the dressing and toss to combine.

Mediterranean Tuna Salad

SERVES 1

6-ounce can albacore tuna, drained and flaked

1 tomato, chopped

½ 15-ounce can chickpeas, drained

1 to 2 tablespoons nonfat Italian dressing

½ cucumber, peeled and cut into chunks

Combine all ingredients in a medium-size bowl and toss to coat with dressing.

Lettuce Shrimp Wrap

SERVES 1

¼ pound cooked shelled rock shrimp
¼ cup chopped celery
¼ cup chopped canned water chestnuts
2 to 3 tablespoons Asian dressing
3 leaves Boston lettuce

Combine the shrimp, celery, and water chestnuts in a medium-size bowl. Use a purchased Asian dressing or make your own using 1 tablespoon honey, 1 tablespoon soy sauce, 1 tablespoon plain rice wine vinegar, and ½ clove garlic, chopped. Add the dressing to the shrimp mixture and toss to combine. Spoon the shrimp mixture into the lettuce leaves and fold to enclose filling.

Zucchini, Sun-Dried Tomato, and Ricotta Tart

SERVES 1

½ small zucchini, finely chopped

4 to 5 sun-dried tomatoes, finely chopped

2 tablespoons nonfat ricotta cheese

¼ cup nonfat milk

4 egg whites (from carton)

Spray a wide, shallow microwave-safe bowl with canola oil. Add all the ingredients to the bowl and beat lightly to combine. Cover with plastic wrap, venting one side, and microwave on High for 3 to 4 minutes, until egg whites are firm.

Meal 4: Afternoon Snack

A few hours before dinner, eat a good-sized snack to get you through the rest of the day. You can go with the morning snack suggestions or heat up a soup that you may have made (see the dinner recipes). Studies have shown that soup is one of the most filling snacks with relatively few calories, mostly because it's liquid. Additionally, here are some good snack choices:

- Celery with nonfat cream cheese and pickle wrapped in turkey pastrami

- Nonflour toast with nonfat cream cheese, smoked salmon and tomato slice

- Turkey breast slices wrapped around lettuce and green pepper strips, with some nonfat cream cheese

- Brown-rice cake with a slice of Veggie salami, fat-free cheese, and mustard

- Beef, salmon, or turkey jerky with piece of fruit

- Pickled herring with nonfat sour cream

- Celery sticks with nonfat French onion soup cream dip

Thai Egg Strips

SERVES 1

4 egg whites (from carton)
1 shallot, minced
1 scallion, thinly sliced
1 small hot red chili, or to taste, minced
1 tablespoon chopped fresh cilantro

Add all the ingredients to a medium-size bowl and beat lightly to combine. Spray a nonstick frying pan with canola oil spray and place over medium heat. Pour in the egg white mixture and cook until a pancake is formed. Place on a plate and slice into diagonal strips.

Meal 5: Dinner

It's the last meal of the day and, hopefully, if you've eaten the other four, you aren't starved. Stick to the essentials of a lean protein taking up a third to a half the meal (chicken/turkey breast, steak—a small portion with no visible fat—or fish and cook it with just ½ teaspoon olive or canola oil), with vegetables (best way is steaming in the microwave or on the stove, in order to preserve the nutrients), and quality carbohydrates (half a sweet potato, squash, ½ cup wild rice, fresh or frozen cauliflower mashed with nonfat half-and-half, etc.) taking up a third each as well. Otherwise, here are some complete meal recipes that you can whip up in a matter of minutes.

Lemon Salmon

SERVES 1

1 8-ounce can wild rice
1 3-ounce salmon fillet (or any fish fillet)
Seasoning to taste (such as lemon pepper or Mrs. Dash)
1 lemon (whole)

Spoon the rice into a microwave-safe container with a lid.

Place the salmon on top of the rice and cover with seasoning (to form a crust).

Squeeze the lemon juice into the container, slice the lemon, and place the slices around the salmon. Cover and microwave on High for 3 to 5 minutes or until salmon is cooked.

Asian Wraps

SERVES 4

1 pound ground chicken breast

3 shiitake mushrooms, chopped

2 teaspoons chopped fresh chives

2 tablespoons black bean sauce

4 leaves Boston lettuce

Lightly spray a sauté pan with canola oil. Add the ground chicken and cook until browned, stirring to break up meat. Add the mushrooms, chives, and black bean sauce. Serve the warm chicken mixture wrapped in a cool lettuce cup. Spread black bean sauce on wrap if desired.

Fish Stew

SERVES 2

1 15-ounce can tomato vegetable or bean soup (such as
    Amy's or Health Valley soups)
1 6-ounce can white albacore tuna, drained
1 tablespoon grated low-fat Parmesan cheese
½ cup crushed baked black-bean tortilla chips
    (optional)
1 tablespoon hot sauce (e.g., Tabasco) (optional)

Mix the soup and tuna in a microwave-safe bowl. Cover with plastic wrap, venting one side, and microwave on High for 2 to 3 minutes or until hot. Add the Parmesan cheese and, if desired, crushed tortillas. Add the hot sauce to desired level of spiciness.

Chicken Fajitas

SERVES 2

½ cup chopped Spanish onion
½ cup chopped bell pepper (any color)
½ pound skinless, boneless chicken breast
1 packet fajita seasoning
2 no-flour tortillas

Spray a medium-size frying pan with canola oil. Add the onion and sauté over medium heat for 2 minutes to soften. Add the bell pepper, chicken breast, and fajita seasoning. Cook for 3 more minutes. Divide between the tortillas and wrap to enclose filling. (As an option, you can add nonfat cheddar cheese, salsa, shredded lettuce, nonfat sour cream, and/or black beans.)

White Bean and Smoked Turkey Soup

SERVES 4

2 teaspoons minced garlic

1 36-ounce can fat-free chicken broth

2 15-ounce cans great northern beans, drained

8 ounces smoked low-fat turkey

1 teaspoon rosemary

Spray a large microwave-safe bowl with canola oil. Add all the ingredients to the bowl. Cover with plastic wrap, venting on one side. Microwave on High for 4 to 5 minutes until hot and bubbly.

Cioppino

SERVES 2

1 15-ounce can organic tomato soup

½ 15-ounce Great Northern beans, drained

1½ cups frozen rock shrimp, scallops, and calamari

3-ounce tilipia fillet, broken up

Fresh chopped or dry basil, to taste

Spray a large microwave-safe bowl with canola oil. Add all the ingredients to the bowl. Cover with plastic wrap, venting on one side. Microwave on High for 4 to 5 minutes. Stir, re-cover, and microwave on High until seafood is cooked.

Thai Lentil Soup

SERVES 4

6½ cups vegetable stock

1 15-ounce can lentil soup

3 tablespoon green curry paste

1 14.5-ounce can crushed tomatoes

3 to 4 ounces shrimp, cleaned and de-veined with tails
removed

Spray a large microwave-safe bowl with canola oil. Add all the ingredients to the bowl. Cover with plastic wrap, venting on one side. Microwave on High for 4 to 5 minutes. Stir in the shrimp, re-cover, and microwave on High until seafood is heated through.

Franks & Beans Soup

SERVES 4

2 large *Yves* Veggie Dogs, chopped

1 15-ounce can baked beans in tomato sauce (no pork
   fat or sugar added)

Spray a medium-size pot with canola oil spray. Add the
Veggie Dogs and beans and bring to a boil over high heat,
then cover and simmer over low heat for 5 minutes.

The Unlisted Meal: Dessert?

You may opt to have something sweet after lunch or dinner. Rather than sugar and/or fat-laden desserts, use a smaller portion of your morning snack options. You may opt for sugar-free pudding with skim milk or sugar-free Jell-O, or part-skim ricotta cheese mixed with Splenda and extract (vanilla, almond, coconut, lemon).

Otherwise, make up one of these 5-Factor healthy desserts that will satisfy your craving. Remember, for the truly rich dessert, wait until your cheat day on Sunday!

- sugar-free gelatin

- fruit salad (with skin still intact)

- sugar-free, fat-free pudding

- sugar-free popsicles

- bowl of berries

Iced Chocolate Delight

SERVES 2

1 package sugar-free hot chocolate mix
½ cup nonfat milk
2 egg whites (from carton)
1 packet Splenda

Add all ingredients to a blender. Blend until frothy. Pour into a small bowl, cover, and chill before serving.

Berry Slush

SERVES 1

1 cup mixed berries
½ cup cold water
Handful of ice
1 teaspoon fresh lemon juice
1 packet Splenda

Place all ingredients to a blender. Blend until berries are pureed. Pour into a glass and serve.

Mocha Ricotta Delight

SERVES 1

½ cup part-skim ricotta cheese

1 shot espresso

1 tablespoon unsweetened cocoa powder

1 packet Splenda

Place all ingredients to a small bowl and mix to combine. Cover and chill before serving.

A FEW THINGS TO TAKE WITH YOU
INTO YOUR 5-FACTOR FUTURE

Now you know how doable and sustainable this program is. You've also read how effective it is. Now the time has come for you to see for yourself. Because the 5-Factor revolves around our typical week cycle, begin the entire program next Monday.

I predict that you're going to get addicted, in a good way, to the workouts and eating style. You will fall in love with the fast workouts, the five meals per day, the variety of it all—and you will wonder how or why, in your quest to get into better shape, you ever tried to go any other way than 5-Factor.

After you get to a place with your body where you are satisfied and pleased, you may modify some parts of the program at certain points. However, because this program doesn't mean arduous changes to your lifestyle, you can keep some form of it in your life for the rest of your life. For example, you may choose to always do the 5-Factor workout and eat five times a day according to most of the meal criteria, yet not keep to every element of the eating program. Whenever you need a tune-up, you can return to the program full-on.

THE MENTAL ESSENTIALS

To ensure short- *and* long-term success on the 5-Factor plan, tune up your mind even before your body.

Look forward, not backward: rather than looking backward and always feeling bad (about the overeating at lunch, the midnight bowl of ice cream, falling off the wagon at your best friend's birthday party, missing workouts on your vacation last week), you have my permission to wipe the slate clean. Start anticipating the next food you're going to put in your mouth and the next workout you're going to do.

Schedule for success: related to the above step, create a basic schedule for five eating times per day (evenly spaced apart) and the five workouts per week. I advocate working out Monday, Tuesday, Thursday, Friday, and Saturday—doing optional cardio on Wednesday and taking Sunday off.

To become fit, *commit:* make the 5-Factor program absolutely fundamental to your present and future health and well-being. Do it not just for yourself, but also for your loved ones. Serve as an inspiration for them.

Say good-bye to flab with *good habits:* make eating and training the 5-Factor way a habit. Try not to miss any workouts, the five meals per day, and the lean protein with each meal, and gradually good eating and exercising will become your natural instinct. When opportunities arise to become lazy or eat terribly, it suddenly will be easier to turn them down. Being healthy and active will soon become automatic.

Learn to love: just as with a successful romantic partnership, being open to discovering new things about working out and eating healthfully will foster a greater bond.

Finally, don't forget to *focus:* our minds can drift off-center—when you're in a restaurant, preparing your dinner, or in the middle of a work-out—if you don't get your head in the present and focus on the essentials at hand (this is as true when you are studying, or even at a religious service). Choose the right foods, savor the flavors—learn to truly relish them—and stick to sensible portions. Use good form with the exercises, breathe with each rep, and give your full effort to the very last rep.

MY FINAL WORDS TO YOU

I'm in my comfort zone when I'm working out—so much so that I'm never happier than when I'm either in the gym or reading about exercise or diet, and when I travel, I choose hotels that have the best gyms.

I understand, though, that you might not share my passion, yet. It may interest you, then, to learn that years ago, I grew frustrated with different exercise programs and eating plans, because they either stopped working for me or were just too hard. Not until the 5-Factor had I found a complete exercise-and-eating plan that not only continued to work for me but that I still *enjoyed* being on. Five years have gone by, and I love the 5-Factor as much as I did that first five weeks. That's the honest truth.

I firmly believe that you, too, will become enamored of this program, once you and those around you see the outstanding results that are waiting for you just around the corner.

So congratulations. In your hands, you have the most efficient, easy-to-use guide to exercise and diet that has ever existed. Now, go on the 5-Factor program for five weeks and see. It could take longer to look like a more fully realized you, but believe me, you'll be well on your way, and you'll have already experienced enormous improvements in your appearance, mental state, energy level, coordination, strength, and confidence. Success truly breeds more success; thus, you'll be able to reach all your fitness goals (and others as well).

I'm excited to see how many of you will make major changes with this program. Send me an e-mail through our website at www.5factorfitness.com and tell me about your success—what you weighed before you started and how your body changed through the course of the program; tell me about how many pounds you lost and how many dress sizes or waist sizes you lost, and what other great changes you experienced in your life. Share your very own 5-Factor recipes. I hope you will tell me that you're still using 5-Factor today.

Note: Italic numbers indicate illustrations.